# CLINICAL SKILLS

## A Nurse's Pocket Guide

# CLINICAL SKILLS
## A Nurse's Pocket Guide

**Rob Schwarz,** MSc, RN

ELSEVIER

London  New York  Oxford  Philadelphia
St Louis  Sydney  Toronto 2022

ELSEVIER

CLINICAL SKILLS: A NURSE'S POCKET GUIDE          ISBN: 978-0-7020-8029-6

### Notice

Practitioners and researchers must always rely on their own experience and knowledge in evaluating and using any information, methods, compounds or experiments described herein. Because of rapid advances in the medical sciences, in particular, independent verification of diagnoses and drug dosages should be made. To the fullest extent of the law, no responsibility is assumed by Elsevier, authors, editors or contributors for any injury and/or damage to persons or property as a matter of products liability, negligence or otherwise, or from any use or operation of any methods, products, instructions, or ideas contained in the material herein.

eISBN 978-0-7020-8030-2

For Elsevier

Content Strategist: Poppy Garraway
Content Development: Veronika Watkins
Project Manager: Julie Taylor
Designer: Amy Buxton

Printed in Scotland

Last digit is the print number:
9  8  7  6  5  4  3  2  1

www.elsevier.com • www.bookaid.org

Working together to grow libraries in developing countries

## CONTENTS

## ACKNOWLEDGEMENTS

This book is dedicated to my wife, Caryl Schwarz, without whose support and kind patience it would not have been possible.

The support and help from my editorial team of Poppy Garraway and Veronika Watkins have been huge in the creation of this book.

The enthusiasm and clarity of thought of my colleague, Kat Johnson, have been immeasurable in pushing this book to completion.

## CHAPTER 1   The Nursing and Midwifery Council (NMC) and the Future of Nursing

- The NMC and this book's purpose
- The NMC document, *Future Nurse: Standards of Proficiency for Registered Nurses 2018*
- The seven platforms
- Annexes A and B

### The NMC and this book's purpose

This book is built around the idea of providing key information in an easy-to-access format that is furnished with explanations and insights that will enable the application and consolidation of fundamental and advanced skills as they are practised.

The conceptual construct that underpins this book is a foundation of three essential purposes: (1) to reflect the NMC document, *Future Nurse: Standards of Proficiency for Registered Nurses 2018* (Nursing and Midwifery Council, 2018), (2) to make information accessible and easy to digest, and (3) to put this text into a pocket-sized book that can be carried into and referenced in the practice environment.

The NMC describes the expected proficiencies of today's modern nurse by organizing them into seven individual platforms.

### The seven platforms

- Being an accountable professional
- Promoting health and preventing ill health
- Assessing needs and planning care
- Providing and evaluating care
- Leading and managing nursing care and working in teams
- Improving safety and quality of care
- Coordinating care

Further to these platforms are two annexes: **Annex A** – Communication and relationship management skills, and **Annex B** – Nursing procedures, which include fundamental nursing skills and also describe the practitioner skills that will facilitate skills of assessment and planning, building to advanced nursing practice.

It is both the core nursing skills and these higher-level practice skills that provide the focus for the content of this book.

### Reference

Nursing and Midwifery Council. (2018). *Future nurse: Standards of proficiency for registered nurses 2018.* London: Nursing and Midwifery Council.

# CHAPTER 2 General Assessment

- First-glance assessment
- Initial actions and MOVE
- ABCDE approach
- NEWS 2 (National Early Warning Score 2)
- SBAR
- Blood pressure, pulse, respiratory rate, temperature
- AVPU
- Fluid balance
- MUST (Malnutrition Universal Screening Tool)
- BMI

## First-glance assessment

When initially assessing a patient, particularly when acute deterioration is suspected, structure your approach along the following lines:
- Is this patient likely to have a respiratory or cardiac arrest imminently?
- How long can I spend assessing before acting?
- What signs can be ascertained immediately?
- What other information is available now?
- What more information can be obtained?
- Do I put out a Medical Emergency Team (MET)/emergency 'crash' call?

Remember, it is OK to put out a crash call even though the patient has not as yet suffered a cardiac or respiratory arrest. The resuscitation of a peri-arrest patient invariably has a better outcome than that of an arrested patient (Schwarz 2006).

## When called to an emergency

- Approach the patient. If the patient is potentially in extremis but showing signs of life, hold the patient's hand, feeling radial pulse. Speak to the patient.
- From this approach you can see if the patient is cold to the touch, potentially peripherally shutting down.
- Is the pulse weak, potentially showing poor pulse volume due to reduced circulatory volume?
- Is the pulse irregular or particularly fast or slow?
- Is the patient breathless? Can they talk in full sentences?
- Is the patient confused, or agitated?
- Whilst this first-glance assessment is happening, ask for the patient's clinical record.

From this initial assessment you can ascertain how urgent the issue is, and potentially from what system the problem is mediated. At this stage a plan should be forming, a plan that is prioritized on urgency of action and focused on further investigation.

## ABCDE assessment

This approach gives the opportunity for an assessment that moves through each area in order of priority, stopping when a problem is found and initiating a process of resolution.

## A = Airway

- Ensure the patient has a patent airway.
- Is the patient talking?
- Is there reduced level of consciousness that may cause an airway obstruction?
- If there is snoring or gasping noises, this may indicate upper airway obstruction.
- Open the airway if necessary using head tilt, chin lift.
- Protect the cervical spine with jaw thrust if cervical injury is suspected.
- Reassess using Look, Listen and Feel technique.
- Secure airway, if at all necessary, using airway adjuncts such as oropharyngeal airway or, if necessary, organize rapid intubation.
- Note paradoxical (see-saw) chest movement, which may indicate a blocked airway.

## B = Breathing

- Assess breathing: rate, rhythm, and depth and efficacy.
- Listen for adventitious respiratory noise such as snoring or wheezing.
- Look for accessory muscles of respiration being used.
- Note symmetry of the chest.
- Is trachea central or deviated?
- Signs of distress, inability to complete sentences.
- Auscultate and percuss if clinical urgency allows.
- Give oxygen if compromised – in an emergency, give high-flow oxygen via a non-rebreather mask. (Once stabilized, titrate the oxygen.)
- Perform pulse oximetry.

## C = Circulation

- Palpate the carotid pulse.
- Look for signs of poor perfusion such as cold extremities, possible confusion, lowered blood pressure, poor pulse volume.
- Note rate and volume of each beat.
- Look for signs of shock.
- Look for signs of haemorrhage.
- Conduct capillary refill time (CRT) by compressing nail bed for 5 seconds and timing the returning blood, which should be less than 2 seconds.
- Measure blood pressure.
- Note temperature.

## D = Disability

- Does the patient have a known medical problem?
- Are there obvious signs of head injury such as the context of collapse (e.g. an obvious fall from a ladder)?
- Is there anyone in attendance who can give a history?
- Measure pupil size and reaction.
- Measure blood glucose level (BGL).
- Assess level of consciousness using AVPU.

  **A Alert**
  **V** Responds to **verbal** stimuli
  **P** Responds to **pain**
  **U Unresponsive**

If response is less than alert, proceed to Glasgow Coma Scale:
- Check drug chart
- Pain score (e.g. numerical rating scale)

## E = Exposure

- Remove the patient's clothing to examine further.
- Be mindful of exposure and hypothermia.
- At all times respect patient's privacy and dignity, and cover when possible.

(RCUK 2015)

## First steps in the deteriorated patient

### Move

**M = Monitor:** Instigate cardiac monitoring. Observe all signs for further deterioration.

**O = Oxygen** is indicated in most peri-arrest situations. Administer high-flow oxygen. Caution should be taken in patients who are known to retain carbon dioxide.

**V = Venous access:** If the patient proceeds to cardiac arrest, establishing access ahead of time will be an invaluable intervention.

**E = ECG & Expert help:** An ECG is a useful intervention even if the problem is not cardiac-mediated, as other problems can be identified, such as electrolyte imbalance, for example.

(RCUK 2015)

## National Early Warning Score (NEWS) 2

The National Early Warning Scoring (NEWS) 2 system (Fig. 2.1) is an approach that was initially developed by the Royal College of Physicians in 2012 and has been updated in 2017. It has been adopted by NHS England as an approved approach to the assessment of the acuity of illness. The way the system works is to collate physiological measurements that are already recorded in clinical practice, which are then given a scoring, with the aggregate of the collective score being used to direct subsequent care. The benefit of the system is that it standardizes the outcome of an assessment and allows acuity to be quickly understood. This is achieved without great workload overhead, in that these observations will be available as part of routine assessments (Royal College of Physicians 2017a).

*Interpretation and triggers for action in NEWS2 (Fig. 2.2)*

*Limitation of NEWS2 scoring system.* Whilst the benefits of the NEWS2 scoring system are obvious, it must be remembered that this process complements clinical judgement and the invaluable tacit insight of the nurse. It must also be remembered that some of the parameters that indicate risk may in fact be steady state or normal observation in some patient groups. For example, a low pulse may be found in the athletic and extremely fit patient and will not indicate a cause for concern; similarly a patient receiving beta-blocker medication may have a pulse below 60, which may be a norm for them that has been therapeutically achieved, which again would have to be considered against the context of a scoring system that has defined this as a risk.

The nature of systematizing a process is that the human engagement can be modified, in that the nurse can be overly reliant on the outcome of this scoring system and either doubt their own insights, if at odds with the defined risk, or indeed inadvertently suspend their clinical oversight.

**Fig. 2.1 The NEWS2 scoring system.** (Royal College of Physicians. (2017). National Early Warning Score (NEWS2) [online]. Available at: https://www.rcplondon.ac.uk/projects/outputs/national-early-warning-score-news-2.)

| Physiological parameter | Score | | | | | | |
|---|---|---|---|---|---|---|---|
| | 3 | 2 | 1 | 0 | 1 | 2 | 3 |
| Respiration rate (per minute) | ≤8 | | 9–11 | 12–20 | | 21–24 | ≥25 |
| SpO₂ Scale 1 (%) | ≤91 | 92–93 | 94–95 | ≥96 | | | |
| SpO₂ Scale 2 (%) | ≤83 | 84–85 | 86–87 | 88–92 ≥93 on air | 93–94 on oxygen | 95–96 on oxygen | ≥97 on oxygen |
| Air or oxygen? | | Oxygen | | Air | | | |
| Systolic blood pressure (mmHg) | ≤90 | 91–100 | 101–110 | 111–219 | | | ≥220 |
| Pulse (per minute) | ≤40 | | 41–50 | 51–90 | 91–110 | 111–130 | ≥131 |
| Consciousness | | | | Alert | | | CVPU |
| Temperature (°C) | ≤35.0 | | 35.1–36.0 | 36.1–38.0 | 38.1–39.0 | ≥39.1 | |

5

| NEW score | Clinical risk | Response |
|---|---|---|
| Aggregate score 0–4 | Low | Ward-based response |
| Red score<br>Score of 3 in any individual parameter | Low–medium | Urgent ward-based response* |
| Aggregate score 5–6 | Medium | Key threshold for urgent response* |
| Aggregate score 7 or more | High | Urgent or emergency response** |

*Response by a clinician or team with competence in the assessment and treatment of acutely ill patients and in recognizing when the escalation of care to a critical care team is appropriate.

**The response team must also include staff with critical care skills, including airway management.

**Fig. 2.2** NEWS2 thresholds and triggers. (Royal College of Physicians. (2017b). National Early Warning Score (NEWS2) [online]. Available at: https://www.rcplondon.ac.uk/projects/outputs/national-early-warning-score-news-2.)

A further concern is that a scoring of NEWS where a full set of observations has not been achieved will distort the aggregate score, so it is important that all staff are aware of the importance of a full set of observations being performed.

A further potential weakness of this system is that a normal score, or a scoring that is defined as risk, could, when viewed over a period of time, in fact, indicate deterioration—for example, a blood pressure that has fallen over a period but currently sits within a range that does not elicit a score indicating risk. Therefore, good practice is to consider NEWS2 scoring against trends over time to ensure that a correct understanding is achieved at all times.

NEWS2 was formally adopted in 2017; this enhancement of the NEWS system was to include elements that enable a broader range of surveillance and give a greater focus on those elements that may indicate the systemic effect of sepsis.

These are:

- A refinement on the oximetry observation, noting use of oxygen therapy and guidance of oxygenation in patients with hypercapnic respiratory failure, namely and most often caused by COPD.
- Greater focus on acute changes in neurological status with AVPU modified to CVPU, where confusion, particularly new onset, is identified as a key indication of increased risk.
- These changes have helped with a particular focus on sepsis, which is a significant problem in the UK and is a leading cause of death. In 2014 there were 123,000 cases with 37,000 deaths, and it is thought that at least 10,000 of these deaths could be avoided with good surveillance and prompt management.

## Sbar

SBAR is an acronym for **S**ituation, **B**ackground, **A**ssessment, **R**ecommendation (Fig. 2.3); this process of structured communication was modified from military use for use in the healthcare setting.

It is a technique that can be used to facilitate prompt and appropriate communication. This communication model is used increasingly in healthcare settings, especially amongst professionals such as physicians and nurses. It is a way for healthcare professionals to communicate effectively with one another, and also allows for important information to be transferred accurately. The format of SBAR allows for short, organized and predictable flow of information between professionals (Uhm et al 2019).

## Blood pressure (BP)

Blood pressure (BP) is two measurements: systole, which is a measure of the pressure exerted by contraction of the heart muscle; and diastole, which is a measure of the pressure when the heart is at the rest stage (Dougherty et al 2015).

## Vital signs and normal values

| | Normal values | Notes |
|---|---|---|
| Temperature | Orally: 36.8°C<br>Tympanic: 37.1–37.4°C<br>Rectal: 37.1–37.4°C<br>Axillary: 35.9–36.7°C | Tympanic is preferred route as most accurate<br>Rectal is considered an invasive procedure<br>Axillary temperature can give a significantly lower reading |
| Pulse (bpm) | 55–90 | A pulse can be lowered if the patient is taking beta-blocker medication<br>The extremely fit patient such as a marathon runner may have non-pathological lower than normal pulse rate<br>Also note rhythm where the heart is beating irregularly<br>Pulse volume is an assessment of the strength of the wave of pressure that is in fact the pulse. Poor pulse volume is likely in low blood pressure or poor cardiac output. Pulse volume can be missed if palpation is not undertaken |
| Respiratory rate | 12–18 breaths per minute | In the adult at rest |
| Blood pressure | 120/70 | Further information on blood pressure below |
| O₂ saturation | 95%–100% | Most pulse oximeters will also give a pulse value |

***Mean arterial pressure.*** The measured fluctuation of pressure within a normal cycle of contraction of the heart will not necessarily indicate the effectiveness of that BP in perfusion of the body's organs; a more exacting measure for this insight is a measurement of mean arterial pressure (MAP).

MAP is most commonly achieved through automated calculation on invasively monitored BP; however. it can be calculated by multiplying the diastolic recording by 2, adding that to the systolic measurement. and then dividing by 3.

$$\text{Diastolic} \times 2 + \text{Systolic} \div 3 = \text{MAP}$$

MAP should be at a minimum of 60 mm Hg to adequately perfuse the body organs.

***Good practice when measuring BP.*** When undertaking BP recording it is important to ensure the correct cuff size is selected, as the wrong size can give an erroneous reading.

When interpreting BP recording it is important to know the norm for the individual patient, as a BP within what would be considered a normal range may be

| S | **Situation:**<br>I am (name), (X) nurse on ward (X)<br>I am calling about (patient X)<br>I am calling because I am concerned that...<br>(e.g. BP is low/high, pulse is XX temperature is XX,<br>Early Warning Score is XX) |
| --- | --- |
| B | **Background:**<br>Patient (X) was admitted on (XX date) with<br>(e.g. MI/chest infection)<br>They have had (X operation/procedure/investigation)<br>Patient (X)'s condition has changed in the last (XX mins)<br>Their last set of obs were (XX)<br>Patient (X)'s normal condition is...<br>(e.g. alert/drowsy/confused, pain free) |
| A | **Assessment:**<br>I think the problem is (XXX)<br>And I have...<br>(e.g. given $O_2$/analgesia, stopped the infusion)<br>OR<br>I am not sure what the problem is but patient (X)<br>is deteriorating<br>OR<br>I don't know what's wrong but I am really worried |
| R | **Recommendation:**<br>I need you to...<br>Come to see the patient in the next (XX mins)<br>AND<br>Is there anything I need to do in the meantime<br>(e.g. stop the fluid/repeat the obs) |

Ask receiver to repeat key information to ensure understanding

The SBAR tool originated from the US Navy and was adapted for use in healthcare by
Dr M Leonard and colleagues from Kaiser Permanente, Colorado, USA

**Fig. 2.3** Situation, Background, Assessment, Recommendation (SBAR).

low when compared with the individual norm—for example, in the instance of essential hypertension.

#### AVPU (Alert, Verbal, Pain, Unresponsive)

AVPU (Fig. 2.4) is a quick and easy way to estimate a patient's level of consciousness (RCUK 2015).

Remember when assessing using NEWS2 that confusion is also a key finding, specifically if new, and may be indicative of the systemic effect of sepsis. With NEWS2 this acronym changes to CAVPU, with the C standing for confusion.

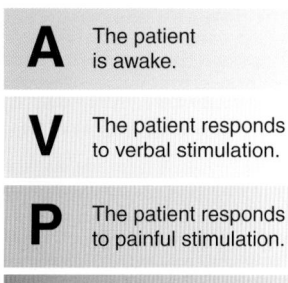

**Fig. 2.4** Alert, Verbal, Pain, Unresponsive (AVPU).

#### Fluid balance

Fluid is constantly leaving the body and, in health, is replaced through diet and fluids; in the therapeutic environment the input may be supplemented with infusions or fluid added to the body in some other manner. When both volumes are equal, it can be said the body is in a fluid balance. Fluid is found in the cells (intracellular), outside the cells (interstitial) and within the blood vessels (intravascular), and whilst fluid moves constantly between these areas, there is an optimum distribution that will enable optimum healthy function of the cells, which is needed to achieve the state of haemostasis (NICE 2013).

    ***Monitoring fluid balance.*** Monitoring fluid balance is essential in many areas of patient care—for example, in cases of renal failure, electrolyte imbalance, vomiting and diarrhea, where fluid drainage is in place, such as nasogastric drainage, and drains from other body cavities.

    When assessing fluid status of a patient there are three elements that need to be observed to create the complete insight; these are the measurement of urinary output, assessment of fluid balance and clinical examination.

    ***Urine output.*** Monitoring urine output is particularly important when assessing fluid balance, and it is usual for a urinary catheter to be used in critical care areas to ensure this is undertaken accurately.

    Urine output should be 0.5–1 mL/kg/hr and when output falls below this threshold it can be indicative of a significant problem.

    Input and output balance should be maintained with cumulative balance over 24 hours, so an ongoing insight into fluid status can be demonstrated.

    With fluid balance it is important to accommodate insensible fluid loss, that is, that fluid which is lost through bodily functions and not measured as fluid. This is fluid lost from the lungs, skin, and respiratory tract, etc., and is thought to be in the range of 800 mL per day for adults.

## Examination

- Skin turgor
- Mucous membrane moistness
- Weight gain over time, typically a day
- Jugular venous pressure (JVP)/central venous pressure (CVP)
- Serum albumin
- Signs of oedema with swollen tissue at the ankles in ambulatory or at the sacrum if bedbound
- Pulmonary oedema will present as breathlessness and as diffuse white opacity on chest X-ray (CXR)

### Skin turgor

Take a small amount of skin between your fingers, rotate gently and watch for a swift return to previous shape. This return suggests elastic properties of the skin which, in turn, can be interpreted as tissue containing an appropriate or high volume of interstitial fluid. This is more difficult to assess in the elderly and may not be as accurate in this patient group.

Moist mucous membrane, typically the tongue, will indicate a good state of hydration; inversely, of course, dry mucous membrane indicates the opposite.

### Jugular venous pressure (JVP)/central venous pressure (CVP)

Fluid can sit in different parts of body tissue and measuring of CVP or examining the jugular veins to estimate venous pressure can give specific information about the venous compartment; when excess fluid sits in the venous compartment it can suggest fluid overload. Remember that veins are compliant and will stretch to accommodate increased volume, whereas the arterial vasculature, having a greater degree of muscle fibre in the vessel wall, will maintain its shape and extra fluid will be demonstrated as an increase in pressure.

The serum proteins, particularly albumin, dictate an osmotic pressure drawing fluid into the blood compartment. So in the instance of lowered albumin, the blood compartment will have a lowered volume with higher volume of fluid in the interstitial places, which will be demonstrated as low BP in the presence of peripheral oedema and weight gain.

*Jugular venous pressure (JVP).* JVP is the indirectly observed pressure in the venous system when viewing the internal jugular vein. An engorged jugular vein can evidence a high venous pressure, when observed in the right context and other extraneous causes are ruled out.

Technique for measuring JVP involves sitting the patient at an angle of 45 degrees and visualizing the internal jugular vein above a level called *the angle of Louis*, which is an imagined straight line from the second pair of costal cartilages to level T4-T5 of the intervertebral discs.

The implication of a high JVP in the context of fluid balance is high venous pressure indicating a high and above-normal volume of fluid in the venous system; this might be found in instances of anuria or oliguria, for example, in renal failure.

*Other causes of elevated JVP*

- Right-sided heart failure
- Pulmonary hypertension

- Tricuspid valve stenosis
- Cardiac tamponade
- Fluid overload as with renal insufficiency or in instances where too much fluid has been infused

*Central venous pressure (CVP).* CVP is the measure of venous pressure through the use of a catheter inserted into the anterior vena cava to the level of the right atrium of the heart, where a transducer can measure venous pressure.

*Causes of raised CVP.* CVP will rise with:
- High venous volume
- Heart failure
- Reduced cardiac output
- Cardiac tamponade

*Low CVP*
- Hypovolaemia
- Distributive shock such as may occur in sepsis or anaphylaxis

## Nutrition

*Malnutrition Universal Screening Tool (MUST) (Fig. 2.5).* (See also Pettit et al 2017.)

*How to Calculate Body Mass Index (BMI)*

$$BMI = \frac{Mass\,(kg)}{Height\,(m)^2}$$

Below 19 = underweight
19–25 = within normal range
25–30 = overweight
30+ = obese

To get the components for the calculation, do the following:
- Measure the patient's height
- Take the patient's weight

For example, a patient of 1.77 m (5 ft 8 in) with a weight of 85 kg would give the following calculation:

Height squared = $1.77 \times 1.77 = 3.13$

Therefore:

$$\frac{85}{3.13} \text{ or } 85 \div 3.13 = 27.15$$

This man's BMI is 27, which is overweight.

Be cautious when using this tool, as it can be inaccurate, particularly if the patient has a lot of muscle mass, which is not differentiated from adipose tissue mass. A further caution is that the tool scores in a very stringent way, and somebody of moderate body mass would be described as overweight with this tool, which in some cases is a very problematic message to give, particularly to young adults in our increasingly body-conscious world.

BAPEN
www.bapen.org.uk

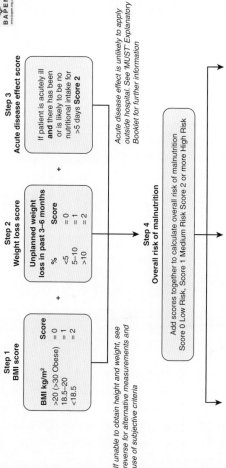

**Step 1**
**BMI score**

| BMI kg/m² | Score |
|---|---|
| >20 (>30 Obese) | = 0 |
| 18.5–20 | = 1 |
| <18.5 | = 2 |

*If unable to obtain height and weight, see reverse for alternative measurements and use of subjective criteria*

+

**Step 2**
**Weight loss score**

**Unplanned weight loss in past 3–6 months**

| % | Score |
|---|---|
| <5 | = 0 |
| 5–10 | = 1 |
| >10 | = 2 |

+

**Step 3**
**Acute disease effect score**

If patient is acutely ill **and** there has been or is likely to be no nutritional intake for >5 days **Score 2**

*Acute disease effect is unlikely to apply outside hospital. See 'MUST' Explanatory Booklet for further information*

**Step 4**
**Overall risk of malnutrition**

Add scores together to calculate overall risk of malnutrition
Score 0 Low Risk, Score 1 Medium Risk Score 2 or more High Risk

13

## Step 5
## Management guidelines

### 0 Low Risk
**Routine clinical care**

- Repeat screening
  Hospital – weekly
  Care Homes – monthly
  Community – annually
  for special groups
  e.g. those >75 yrs

### 1 Medium Risk
**Observe**

- Document dietary intake for 3 days

- If adequate – little concern and repeat screening
  - Hospital – weekly
  - Care Home – at least monthly
  - Community – at least every 2–3 months

- If inadequate – clinical concern – follow local policy, set goals, improve and increase overall nutritional intake, monitor and review care plan regularly

### 2 or more High Risk
**Treat***

- Refer to dietitian, Nutritional Support Team or implement local policy
- Set goals, improve and increase overall nutritional intake
- Monitor and review care plan
  Hospital – weekly
  Care Home – monthly
  Community – monthly

*Unless detrimental or no benefit is expected from nutritional support e.g. imminent death.

### All risk categories:

- Treat underlying condition and provide help and advice on food choices, eating and drinking when necessary.
- Record malnutrition risk category.
- Record need for special diets and follow local policy.

### Obesity:

- Record presence of obesity. For those with underlying conditions, these are generally controlled before the treatment of obesity.

**Re-assess subjects identified at risk as they move through care settings**
See *The 'MUST' Explanatory Booklet* for further details and *The 'MUST' Report* for supporting evidence.

**Fig. 2.5** Malnutrition Universal Screening Tool (MUST). (BAPEN. (2020). The 'MUST' Toolkit [online]. Available at: https://www.bapen.org.uk/ screening-and-must/must/must-toolkit/the-must-itself.)

© BAPEN

It should be remembered that BMI is only one tool, and other measures are available (e.g. body fat, arm circumference). However, the BMI measurement is by far the most commonly used and in effect has become, by default, an industry standard.

## References

Dougherty, L., Lister, S., West-Oram, A. (eds). (2015). *The Royal Marsden Manual of Clinical Nursing Procedures*. Student Edition. (9th ed.). Chichester: Wiley-Blackwell.

Pettit, J., James, J., Gilby, L. (2017). Delivering NoSH (Nutritional Support in Hospital): Support for nutrition in hospital. *Journal of Dementia Care*, 25(3), 22–24.

Resuscitation Council (UK) (RCUK). (2015). *The ABCDE approach*. London: Resuscitation Council (UK).

Royal College of Nursing. (2017). *Standards for assessing, measuring and monitoring vital signs in infants, children and young people: RCN guidance for nurses working with children and young people*. London: Royal College of Nursing (RCN).

Royal College of Physicians. (2017b). *National Early Warning Score (NEWS) 2*. Working party report. London: Royal College of Physicians (RCP).

Schwarz, R. (2006). Beginner to Specialist (1st ed.). Essential Knowledge Publishing Limited, UK.

Uhm, J.Y., Ko, Y., Kim, S. (2019). Implementation of an SBAR communication program based on experiential learning theory in a paediatric nursing practicum: A quasi-experimental study. *Nurse Education Today*, 80, 78–84.

## Further Reading

Cross, R., Considine, J., Currey, J. (2019). Nursing handover of vital signs at the transition of care from the emergency department to the inpatient ward: An integrative review. *Journal of Clinical Nursing*, 28(5–6), 1010–1021.

Grant, S. (2018). Limitations of track and trigger systems and the National Early Warning Score. Part 1: Areas of contention. *British Journal of Nursing*, 27(11), 624–631.

Health Service Executive, Republic of Ireland. (2019). *Implementation toolkit for the food, nutrition and hydration policy for adult patients in acute hospitals*. Dublin: Health Service Executive, Republic of Ireland.

Müller, M., et al. (2018). Impact of the communication and patient hand-off tool SBAR on patient safety: a systematic review. *BMJ*, 8(8), e022202.

NHS England. (2018). Taking on a silent killer: a systematic approach. Available at: https://www.england.nhs.uk/rightcare/2018/06/19/taking-on-a-silent-killer-a-system-approach/

National Institute for Health and Care Excellence (NICE). (2013). *Intravenous fluid therapy in adults in hospital*. Clinical guideline [CG174]. London: NICE.

National Institute for Health and Care Excellence (NICE). (2006). *Nutrition support for adults: oral nutrition support, enteral tube feeding and parenteral nutrition*. Clinical guideline. [CG32] London: NICE.

Royal College of Physicians. (2017a). *Improving teams in healthcare: Resource 3 – team communication*. London Royal College of Physicians (RCP).

## CHAPTER 3 Airway

- Head tilt, chin lift
- Jaw thrust
- Oropharyngeal airway
- Nasopharyngeal airway
- Bag valve mask
- Choking

Since 2005 there has been an emphasis on chest compression as a priority above respiratory support, as it has been recognized that adult cardiac arrest is mediated by a cardiac event, in most cases, which means that respiratory function has been intact until that point. The implication of this insight is that the blood is likely to be well oxygenated, and moving this oxygenated blood with chest compressions is the most expeditious way to preserve vulnerable tissues of the brain and heart. However, opening the airway and giving ventilation support is a key intervention once chest compression resuscitation is established (RCUK 2021; Nolan, J., Soar, J., Eikeland, H., 2006).

To open the airway of the unconscious patient there are two methods:
- Head tilt, chin lift (Fig. 3.1)
- Jaw thrust (Fig. 3.2), which keeps the cervical spine in alignment if there is risk of instability due to cervical fracture, which in turn puts the cervical spine at risk

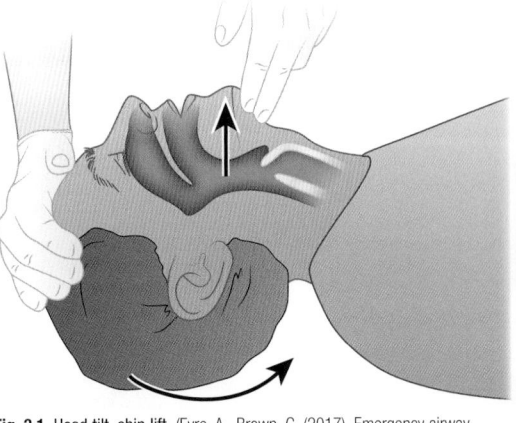

**Fig. 3.1** Head tilt, chin lift. (Eyre, A., Brown, C. (2017). Emergency airway management. In: P. Auerbach (ed) Auerbach's Wilderness Medicine (7th edn) (pp. 403–419). Philadelphia: Elsevier.)

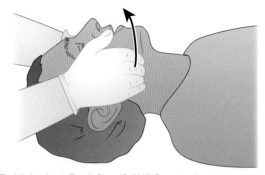

**Fig. 3.2** Jaw thrust. (Eyre, A., Brown, C. (2017). Emergency airway management. In: P. Auerbach (ed) Auerbach's Wilderness Medicine (7th edn) (pp. 403–419). Philadelphia: Elsevier.)

## Assessment with the look, listen and feel technique

Assessment of the airway is achieved with the Look, Listen and Feel approach (Fig. 3.3), where the rescuer:

- **Looks** for chest movement
- **Listens** for breath sounds
- **Feels** for the movement of breath against the cheek (Resuscitation Council (UK) (RCUK)., 2013

## Airway management: Next steps

Airway adjuncts can be used to consolidate the airway when the patient is unconscious and unable to do so himself; whilst these help to improve patency of the airway, they do not definitively protect it.

### The oropharyngeal airway

The oropharyngeal airway (Fig. 3.4) is a plastic tube curved and shaped to fit between the tongue and the hard palate. While not a definitively secured airway, it is useful particularly in the resuscitation scenario as it stops soft palate obstruction and backward displacement of the tongue. When using this airway adjunct, the airway manoeuvres of head tilt, chin lift or jaw thrust may also be needed.

Sizing of the oropharyngeal airway is important as an incorrectly sized airway can in fact cause obstruction itself. To correctly size the airway, place the airway beside the patient's face, aligning the mouth guard to the unconscious patient's incisors so that the end of the airway reaches down to the angulation of the mandible. If the airway meets these two anatomical points, this can be said to be the correct size.

The oropharyngeal airway is inserted with the curved tip pointing to the roof of the mouth and as the airway is advanced it is rotated. This technique allows

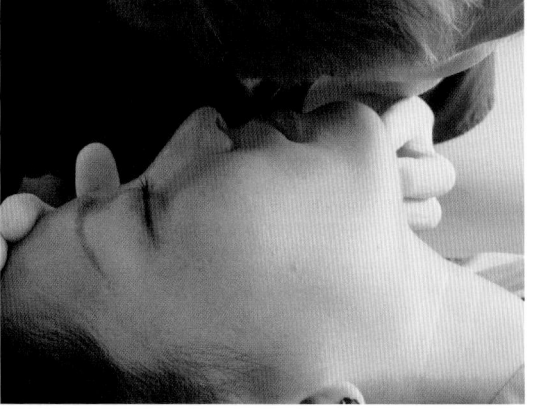

**Fig. 3.3** Assessment with Look, Listen and Feel. (Malamed, S. (2018). Sedation: a guide to patient management (6th edn) (pp. 380–398). St. Louis: Elsevier.)

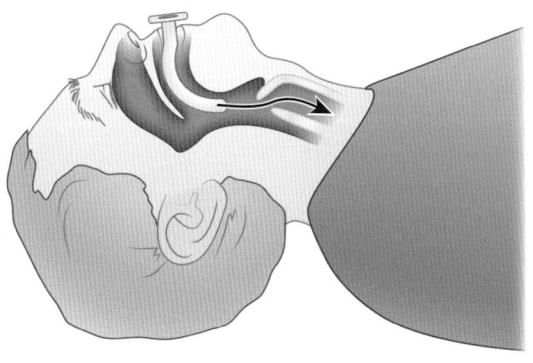

**Fig. 3.4** The oropharyngeal airway. (Eyre, A., Brown, C. (2017). Emergency airway management. In: P. Auerbach (ed) Auerbach's Wilderness Medicine (7th edn) (pp. 403–419). Philadelphia: Elsevier.)

placement over the tongue and prevents pushing the tongue back over the patient's airway.

Following insertion, patency should be checked by inflating the patient's lungs and assessing using the Look, Listen and Feel method or auscultation of the chest listening for air movement.

### The nasopharyngeal airway

The nasopharyngeal airway (Fig. 3.5) is a malleable tube inserted via the nostril and sits in the same space as the oropharyngeal airway. It is better tolerated than the oropharyngeal airway and can be used when there are issues mobilizing the jaw, such as trismus, clenched jaw or injuries in this area.

Sizing is achieved comparing the diameter of the tube against the patient's little finger, as the diameter increases with length. Care should be taken in use with patients who have suffered a base of skull fracture, as there has been instance of the airway being inserted into the cranial vault. Once the airway is in place a safety pin should be inserted across the base of the tube to ensure it remains in place.

### Bag valve mask

Bag valve mask (Fig. 3.6) is a key piece of equipment in resuscitation and is used to enable manual positive pressure ventilation. The three component parts give the equipment its name. The mask is a hard plastic cone-shaped mask with an inflatable soft cushion edge, which enables a seal when pressure is applied. The valve connects the mask to the bag reservoir and allows the passage of oxygen-enriched air when pressure is applied to the bag and allows expired air to be released to the atmosphere. The bag is the third part of the equipment, and allows the movement

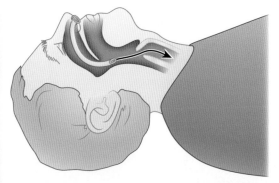

**Fig. 3.5** The nasopharyngeal airway. (Eyre, A., Brown, C. (2017). Emergency airway management. In: P. Auerbach (ed) Auerbach's Wilderness Medicine (7th edn) (pp. 403–419). Philadelphia: Elsevier.)

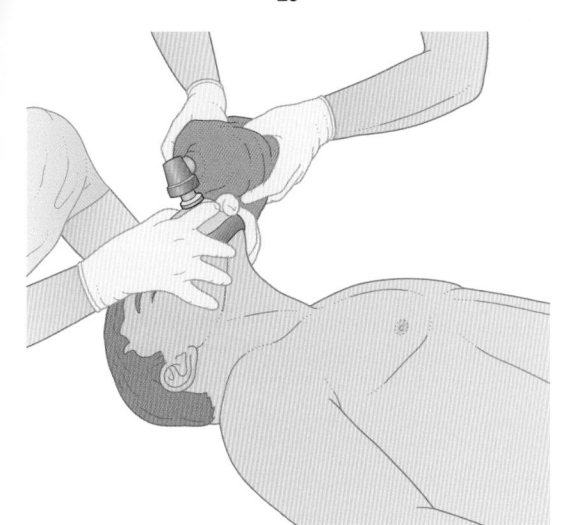

**Fig. 3.6** Bag valve mask. (Freeman, J. (2018). Cardiopulmonary resuscitation. In: H. Stein, R. Stein, M. Freeman (eds), The ophthalmic assistant (10th edn) (pp. 750–762). Elsevier.)

of oxygenated air under manual pressure when the bag is squeezed. This equipment is most effectively used as a two-person manoeuvre, with one holding the mask to the patient's face, creating a seal, whilst the second applies the intermittent compression of the bag reservoir; this is done at a rate of 10–12 per minute, with oxygen tubing attached and delivering oxygen at a rate of 10 litres, which delivers the ventilation breath enriched to 85% oxygen.

## Choking algorithm (Fig. 3.7)

### The back blows

When delivering back slaps, use one hand to support the patient whilst bending them forward and then deliver the back blow with a full hand directed between the shoulder blades. The blow should be delivered with some force, remembering that this is a life-saving manoeuvre.

The abdominal thrust is achieved by bringing the fist of the hand up to the top of the patient's abdomen, with the other hand of the rescuer placed over the first hand and then, with the patient bent forward slightly, the fist is pulled back and up in an assertive and quick way.

**Adult choking**

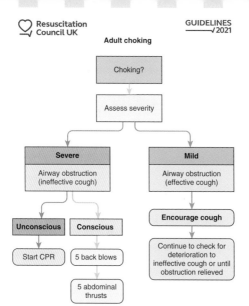

**Fig. 3.7** Choking algorithm. (Resuscitation Council (UK). (2021). *Adult choking algorithm*. London: Resuscitation Council (UK).)

For the bed-bound patient, back slaps and the abdominal thrust should still be attempted and where unconsciousness occurs move on to CPR even in the presence of a palpable pulse, as the rationale for this action is to try and dislodge the obstruction by actions of chest compression applying upward pressure and ventilation providing downward pressure. The purpose of both actions is to move the obstruction in any or either direction, and if the obstruction moves toward the lung it will move into the right main bronchus, allowing the left lung to ventilate and thereby saving a life (Dougherty, L., Lister, S., West-Oram, A., 2015; Resuscitation Council UK RCUK., 2021).

## References

Dougherty, L., Lister, S., West-Oram, A. (eds). (2015). *The Royal Marsden Manual of Clinical Nursing Procedures. Student Edition.* (9th ed.). Chichester: Wiley-Blackwell.

Nolan, J., Soar, J., Eikeland, H. (2006). The chain of survival. *Resuscitation*, 71(3), 270–271.

Resuscitation Council (UK) (RCUK). (2013). *Quality standards for cardiopulmonary resuscitation practice and training.* London: Resuscitation Council (UK). Available at: https://www.resus.org.uk/library/quality-standards-cpr

Resuscitation Council (UK) (RCUK). (2021). *Resuscitation Guidelines 2021: Adult advanced life support.* London: Resuscitation Council (UK).

## CHAPTER 4 Breathing (Respiratory Assessment)

- Chest auscultation
- Normal/abnormal sounds
- Oxygen therapy
- Chest X-ray analysis (10-point analysis process, requesting the CXR)
- Arterial blood gas interpretation

## Examining the chest

The examination of the chest has become a key skill for the nurse, and is one of the NMC expected proficiencies of the standards for the newly qualified staff nurse (NMC 2018).

### The first approach to the patient – the first glance assessment

On first glance, note the following:
- Breathlessness
- Inability to complete full sentences
- Accessory muscles in use
- Unequal expansion of the chest wall
- Little or poor effort
- Audible wheeze
- Upper respiratory tract noise, such as stridor

### Chest auscultation

#### Prepare the environment
- Create as quiet an environment as possible
- Patient should be sitting up with nothing leaning against their chest
- Stethoscope should touch the patient's bare skin
- One can wet chest hair to decrease sounds caused by friction where the hair makes contact with the stethoscope

#### When listening
- Use the diaphragm of the stethoscope
- Ask the patient not to speak
- Ask the patient to breathe deeply through the mouth
- Listen to one full breath at each location
- Compare side to side

#### Chest auscultation (Fig. 4.1)

There are 12–14 auscultation sites on the anterior and posterior, respectively – listen to at least 12 locations.

Start at the apices, working side to side and down to bases. If there is a suspicious sound, listen to nearby locations to assess extent and character.

Locations are organized into categories based on intensity, pitch location and character.

Sounds are created by turbulent airflow. Expiratory breath sounds are quieter than inspiratory as the sound is going toward larger airways.

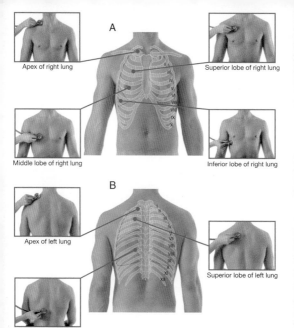

**Fig. 4.1** Chest auscultation. **A**, Anterior view. **B**, Posterior view. (Drake, R., Vogl, W., Mitchell, A. (2018). Thorax. In: *Gray's Basic Anatomy* (2nd edn) (pp. 57–132). Philadelphia: Elsevier.)

### Normal sounds

*Tracheal or bronchial*
- Heard over trachea and main stem bronchus
- Loud and high pitched
- Heard over anterior chest wall, second to fourth intercostal space (ICS) and third to sixth posterior

*Vesicular*
- Heard over the thorax, therefore most of the lung
- Soft and low pitched
- Inspiratory sound longer than expiratory

*Bronchovesicular*
- Best heard over the first and second ICS (anterior chest) and between the scapulae (posterior chest)
- Pitch and duration between vesicular and bronchial

**Abnormal breath sounds**
- Bronchial breath sounds in wrong location
- Louder than normal breath sounds
- Heard when bronchi open into consolidated tissue, for example pneumonia
- Remember consolidated tissue will transmit noise more effectively then tissue filled with air.

**Diminished breath sounds.** Diminished breath sounds can be a normal finding; however, they may be secondary to increased sound filtration due to anomalous features such as pleural effusion or thickening of tissue. Breath sounds will diminish when there is decreased chest movement with decreased air movement.

Possible causes of diminished breath sounds:
- Emphysema
- Severe asthma
- Pneumothorax
- Atelectasis
- Pleural effusion
- Acute respiratory distress syndrome (ARDS) in later stages

**Absent breath sounds when found regionally: causes**
- Pneumothorax: this, when found, is a medical emergency and needs immediate action
- Pleural effusion
- Atelectasis (adjacent tracheal sounds may be heard in auscultation of upper right lobe where atelectasis is defined)

**Adventitious breath sounds.** Adventitious sounds are not abnormal breath sounds but rather sounds that have been added to normal breath sounds.
- Not heard over normal healthy lungs
- Heard from lungs, pleura or pericardium
- Can be discontinuous or contiguous

*Wheezes*
- Continuous high-pitched musical sound
- Produced when air flows through airways narrowed by secretions, foreign bodies or obstructive lesions
- Monophonic (one airway affected) or polyphonic (generalized obstruction)
- Can be found on inspiration, expiration
- Have a longer duration than crackles
- May clear on coughing

Wheezes at the mouth and breath sounds absent or substantially diminished signify significant severity and may proceed to respiratory arrest.

*Causes*
- Asthma
- Chronic bronchitis
- Chronic obstructive pulmonary disease (COPD)
- Congestive cardiac failure

- Pulmonary oedema
- Foreign body
- Mucosal swelling as found in anaphylaxis
- Tumour

### Stridor

- Stridor is a medical emergency – intubation or tracheotomy may be indicated
- Loud musical monophasic wheeze
- Often heard without stethoscope
- Intensity distinguishes it from other monophasic wheezes
- Usually inspiratory but can be heard throughout respiratory cycle as airway constriction increases

#### Causes

- Anaphylaxis
- Sever upper airway respiratory infection
- Laryngeal tumours
- Tracheal stenosis
- Whooping cough
- Aspiration of foreign body

### Pleural rub

- When the pleural surfaces are inflamed or roughened and move against each other
- Creaking or brushing sound
- Discontinuous or continuous
- Can be localized to a particular place on the chest wall
- Heard at both inspiration and expiration

#### Causes

- Pleural effusion
- Pneumothorax

### Crackles or crepitations

- Sounds like hair being rubbed together
- Non-musical sounds more commonly heard on inspiration

There are two explanations of how these noises are created. The first is that small airways open during inspiration but collapse during expiration causing the crackle. The second explanation is that air bubbles travel through secretions or partly closed airways during expiration causing this noise (Heuer & Scanlan 2017).

---

### Chest auscultation key points

- Findings can be normal breath sounds, abnormal breath sounds or adventitious sounds
- Any crackles will alert you to a problem
- Always find out a patient's medical history
- Use chest auscultation as an adjunct to overall diagnosis

### Arterial blood gases (ABGs)

- When interpreting ABGs, one needs to consider the nature of the chemicals being measured; if you know the characteristics of these chemicals, you can anticipate what effect they will have on the patient's physiology.

- Carbon dioxide ($CO_2$) is a gas dissolved in blood, that is acid in its nature and therefore at high levels it can make the blood acidic. A high $CO_2$ level equates to acidosis. The other thing that is known about $CO_2$ is that it is a by-product of respiration; when found in high quantities, the cause is related to respiration.
- Bicarbonate ($HCO_3$) is a chemical that buffers acid, and this process uses up $HCO_3$ causing its levels to fall in acidosis; in alkalosis the opposite will happen – $HCO_3$ will rise.
- Acidosis occurs when the pH is below 7.35.
- There are two types of acidosis: respiratory, where high levels of $CO_2$ are found; and metabolic, where low levels of $CO_2$ are found with a concurrent fall in $HCO_3$.
- Alkalosis occur when the pH rises, which can occur with hyperventilation or other disorders that can affect respiration, such as stroke, where the excess breath causes the $pCO_2$ dissolved in the blood to fall. In metabolic alkalosis the bicarbonate in the blood increases, which can be caused by excessive vomiting, nasogastric drainage, hypokalaemia and poorly controlled diuretic use.

## Compensation

Compensation is the natural process where the body tries to maintain the correct pH. There are two systems that come into play to achieve this – the respiratory system and the renal system – and consequently compensation is described as respiratory or renal compensation. The respiratory system will affect pH by regulating the $CO_2$ level, whereas the renal system will effect change through retention of bicarbonate. The respiratory system will come to effect within minutes and achieve maximal effect in 24 hours whereas renal effect begins at 6–12 hours, reaching maximal effect at 3 to 4 days.

## ABGs – normal values

| | |
|---|---|
| pH | 7.35–7.45 |
| PaO$_2$ | 10.8–15.0 kPa |
| PaCO$_2$ | 4.5–6.0 kPa |
| HCO$_3$ | 22–28 mmol/L |
| BE | = 2 to -2 mmol/L |

## Indications for ABGs

ABGs are an invasive procedure that can have serious complications such as infection, extravasation and potentially restriction of blood flow to the hand, so it is important that correct indications for undertaking this procedure are observed. Following are likely situations warranting ABG sampling:
- Respiratory failure
- COPD, particularly in exacerbation
- Undiagnosed severe respiratory illness
- Any illness where metabolic acidosis might be a concern, such as cardiac failure, liver failure, renal failure
- Diabetes, particularly ketoacidosis
- Patients receiving respiratory support in the form of ventilation and NIPPY, when used in acute illness

**Blood gas analysis**

| Acid base disorder | pH | $CO_2$ | $HCO_3$ |
|---|---|---|---|
| Respiratory acidosis | ↓ | ↑ | N |
| Metabolic acidosis | ↓ | N | ↓ |
| Respiratory alkalosis | ↑ | ↓ | N |
| Metabolic alkalosis | ↑ | N | ↑ |
| Respiratory acidosis with renal compensation | ↓ or N | ↑ | ↑ |
| Respiratory alkalosis with renal compensation | ↑ or N | ↓ | ↓ |
| Metabolic acidosis with respiratory compensation | ↓ | ↓ | ↓ |
| Metabolic alkalosis with respiratory compensation | ↑ | ↑ | ↑ |

(RCUK 2021)

## Oxygen therapy

Oxygen administration is an essential treatment in many conditions, particularly the acutely unwell. The purpose of oxygen therapy is to treat hypoxia, and it should be prescribed in accordance with a desired $O_2$ saturation.

The British Thoracic Society guideline states the ideal range as 94%–97%.

Caution should be exercised with the $CO_2$ retention patient, as their pathological drive to breathe is caused by lack of oxygen, and therefore oxygen therapy can repress their respiration.

In an emergency, give high-flow oxygen but observe for adverse effect.

Surveillance of oxygen therapy should include oxygen saturation and noting rate of respiration, type of respiration and accessory muscles being used. With oximetry it is important to ensure that the patient has nothing on the nail bed that might distort the reading, such as nail varnish (Hennessey & Japp 2015).

**Types of oxygen therapy**

| Device | Flow rates litres of oxygen/minute | Delivered oxygen |
|---|---|---|
| Nasal cannula | 1 L/min | 21%–24% |
|  | 2 L/min | 25%–28% |
| Simple oxygen face mask | 6–10 L/min | 35%–60% |
| Venturi mask | 4–8 L/min | 24%–40% |
|  | 10–12 L/min | 40%–50% |
| Non-rebreather mask (face mask with reservoir) | 15 L/min | 80%–95% |

## The chest X-ray

The chest X-ray (CXR) is a common procedure which can give information that is significantly supportive to enable diagnosis. Previously the prerogative of the doctor, it is now becoming more frequently the prerogative of other healthcare professionals and notably nurses, who are now often found requesting and interpreting chest X-rays.

If you are ordering X-rays as part of your role, ensure you are appropriately trained in the management of X-ray radiation. Ionizing Radiation (Medical Exposure) Regulations training, or IR(ME)R, is the recognized course.

## Rationale for ordering CXR

- Necessary as adjunct to diagnosis and treatment
- Exclude respiratory pathology in patients with potentially respiratory-mediated problems
- Confirmation of central venous pressure (CVP) line
- Confirmation of nasogastric (NG) tube placement

## CXR analysis

### Basic analysis

- Patient identity information
- Date and time
- Anterior posterior (AP) or posterior anterior (PA) film
- Technical quality
- Check for rotation: was the patient correctly positioned when the X-ray was taken?

### Assessing technical quality

- Assessing the quality of the X-ray penetration: you should be able to see the lower thoracic vertebral bodies through the heart
- Assessing if the patient is rotated: the spinous process of the thoracic vertebrae should sit midway between the medial ends of the clavicles
- Most X-ray films are taken posterior anterior (PA); that is, the X-ray is taken through the back of the patient towards the X-ray plate at the front
- PA view is considered better as from this position the heart is not magnified as in a AP film

---

### The 10-point CXR analysis approach

**Point 1:** Is there pathology of the bones?
**Point 2:** Is there evidence of pathology of the soft tissue of the chest wall?
**Point 3:** Is the trachea straight?
**Point 4:** Is the heart a normal size? It should be less than half the width of the thorax. If the film is taken AP then it may appear larger.
**Point 5:** Is there mediastinal widening?
**Point 6:** Are the hila pulled up or down? (The left is normally higher than the right.)
**Point 7:** Is the diaphragm raised? (The right is normally higher than the left as it sits over the liver.)
**Point 8:** Are the lung fields clear of shadowing?
**Point 9:** Are the costophrenic angles free of shadowing?
**Point 10:** Is there good inspiration? The diaphragm should lie at the level of the sixth ribs anteriorly.

### CXR analysis – a closer look

- The trachea should be central. (The most common cause of deviation is pneumothorax, which, given the severity of the condition, should be identified and managed clinically and not delayed by seeking X-ray confirmation.)
- The aortic arch is the first structure on the left, followed by the left pulmonary artery, with fanning arterial branches seen extending into the lung.
- Two-thirds of the heart lies on the left side of the chest, with one-third on the right.
- The heart should take no more than a half of the view of the horizontal plane of the base of the thorax.
- Above the right heart border lies the edge of the superior vena cava.
- The pulmonary arteries and main bronchi rise from the left and right hila. Enlarged lymph glands and tumours can occur here, which will make them appear bulky and larger than they should be.
- Now look at each lung, starting at the apex and working down to the bases, comparing left to right as you move down the X-ray.
- The radiotranslucence of the lungs should render them black on X-ray with only pulmonary vessels being seen.
- Actively look for pneumothorax, which will show as a sharp line at the edge of the lung field.
- Make sure you can see the surface of the hemidiaphragms curving downwards and that the costophrenic angles are not blunted, suggestive of effusion or oedema.
- Check there is no air under the hemidiaphragms (Lacey et al 2008).

## References

Hennessey, I., Japp, A. (2015). *Arterial blood gases made easy*. London: Elsevier.

Heuer, A.J., Scanlan, C. (2017). *Clinical assessment in respiratory care*. London: Elsevier.

Lacey, G., Morley, S., Berma, L. (2008). *The chest x-ray: a survival guide* (1st edn). London: Elsevier.

Nursing and Midwifery Council (NMC). (2018). *Future Nurse: Standards of proficiency for registered nurses 2018*. London: Nursing and Midwifery Council.

O'Driscoll, B.R., Howard, L.S., Earis, J., et al; BTS Emergency Oxygen Guideline Development Group on behalf of the British Thoracic Society. (2017). British Thoracic Society Guideline for oxygen use in adults in healthcare and emergency settings. *Thorax*, 72(Supp 1), i1–i90.

Resuscitation Council (UK) (RCUK). (2021). *Resuscitation Guidelines 2021: adult advanced life support*. London: Resuscitation Council (UK).

## Further Reading

Corne, J., Pointon, K. (2010). *Chest X-ray made easy* (3rd edn). London: Churchill Livingstone Elsevier.

Ellis, S. (2010). *Interpreting chest X-rays*. Banbury, UK: Scion Publishing.

Sud, M., Barolet, A., McDonald, M., Floras, J.S. (2013). Anterior crackles: a neglected sign. Canadian *Journal of Cardiology*, 29(9), 11138.e1–e2.

Smeltzer, S.C., Bare, B.G., Hinkle, J.L., Cheever, K.H. (2010). *Brunner and Suddarth's textbook of medical surgical nursing*. Philadelphia: Lippincott Williams & Wilkins.

# CHAPTER 5  Circulation (Cardiovascular Assessment)

- ECG monitoring and taking the ECG
- Five-stage ECG interpretation
- Cardiac arrhythmias
- Auscultation sites
- Heart sounds interpretation

### ECG monitoring lead placement (Fig. 5.1)

**Red** – right arm or second intercostal space on the right of the sternum
**Yellow** – left arm or second intercostal space on the left of the sternum
**Black** or **green** – left leg or more commonly in the region of the apex beat.
This allows lead I, II or III configurations to be selected on the ECG monitor; lead II
is the most commonly used (Hampton 2019).

Electrode
placement

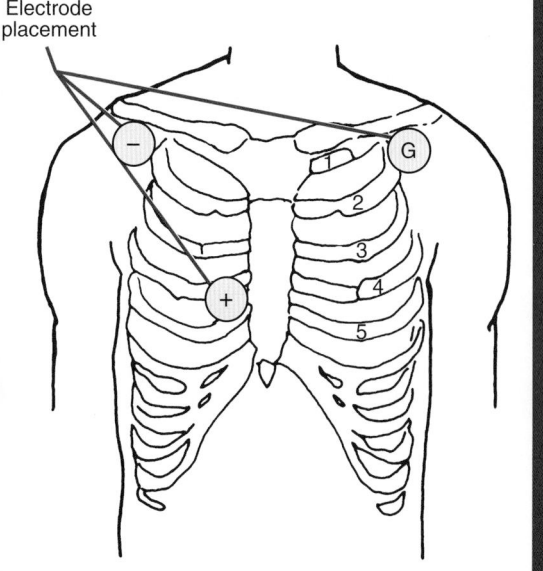

**Fig. 5.1** ECG monitoring lead placement. (Goldberger, A., Goldberger, Z., Shvilkin, A. (2018). ECG leads. In: *Goldberger's Clinical Electrocardiography: A Simplified Approach* (9th edn) (pp. 21–31). Philadelphia: Elsevier.)

## ECG lead placement – chest and limb (Fig. 5.2)

### Five stages of ECG interpretation

1. Rate: What is the QRS rate?
2. Rhythm: Is the QRS rate regular or irregular?
3. Is the QRS width normal or prolonged?
4. Is there atrial activity present indicated by the 'P' wave? Are the 'P' waves normal?
5. What is the relationship between atrial activity and ventricular activity?

## The normal ECG (Fig. 5.3)

**P** = Atrial activity

**QRS** = Ventricular contraction

**T** = Repolarization of the ventricles

**Rate:** To calculate the rate, divide 300 by the number of big squares per 'R' to 'R' interval

**Rhythm:** If it is unclear if a rhythm is regular or not, take a piece of card and mark six 'R' waves and then move the card along to see if the marks match subsequent 'R' waves

**Is QRS widened**? QRS should be narrow 0.08–0.12 seconds (2–3 small squares) The widening of QRS shows a slower spread of ventricular depolarization. Widened QRS is seen with ventricular ectopic beats, in VF, and bundle branch block (BBB).

## Widened QRS

- Is there a 'P' wave (Fig. 5.6)?
- What is the relationship of the "P" wave (atrial activity) and the QRS (ventricular activity)? Does it look normal? Is it the correct distance from the QRS part of the complex? Is there a delay between 'P' wave and the QRS part of the complex? Does the 'P' wave appear within the complex?

## A normal ECG trace (Fig. 5.7)

- Rate is 75 bpm
- The rate is regular; note the constant distance between each 'R' to 'R' interval
- QRS is normal in that it is less than 0.1 second
- The is a 'P' wave before each QRS
- PR interval is normal at less than 0.2 seconds

## Common ECG examples

### Ventricular fibrillation (Fig. 5.8)

Broad complexes, erratic, fast, disordered morphology, difficult to accurately measure, no 'P' waves.

### Ventricular tachycardia (Fig. 5.9)

Broad complexes, fast given disordered morphology, difficult to accurately measure but in the range of 200, no 'P' waves.

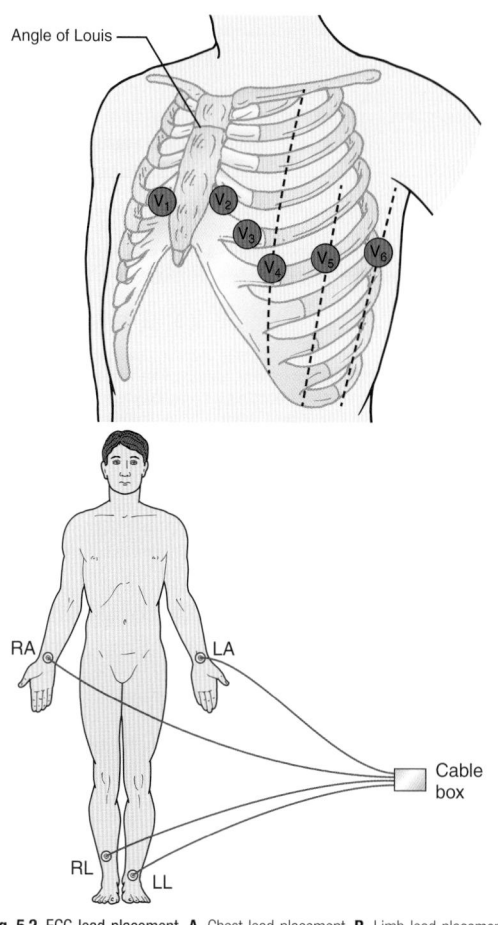

Angle of Louis

$V_1$ $V_2$ $V_3$ $V_4$ $V_5$ $V_6$

RA  LA

RL  LL

Cable box

**Fig. 5.2** ECG lead placement. **A**, Chest lead placement. **B**, Limb lead placement. (Goldberger, A., Goldberger, Z., Shvilkin, A. (2018). ECG leads. In: *Goldberger's Clinical Electrocardiography: A Simplified Approach* (9th edn) (pp. 21–31). Philadelphia: Elsevier.)

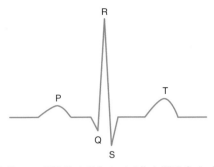

**Fig. 5.3** The normal ECG. (Apple, F., Goetze, J., Jaffe, A. (2018). Cardiac function. In: N. Rifai (ed), *Textbook of clinical chemistry and molecular diagnostics* (6th edn) (pp. 1201–1255). St. Louis, MO: Elsevier.)

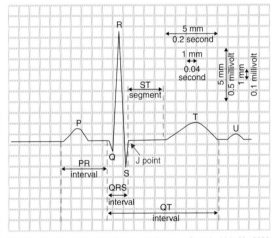

**Fig. 5.4** Inscription of a normal electrocardiogram. (Ganz, L., Link, M., 2020 Electrocardiography. In: L. Goldman, A. Schaffer (eds), *Goldman-Cecil medicine* (26th edn) (pp. 246–253). Philadelphia: Elsevier.)

# QRS Interval

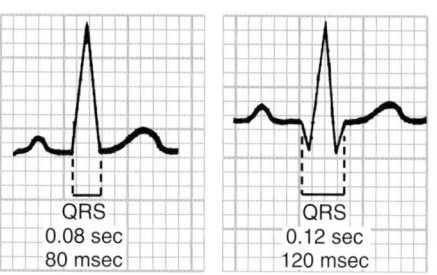

**Fig. 5.5** QRS interval. (Goldberger, A., Goldberger, Z., Shvilkin, A. (2018). How to make basic ECG measurements. In: *Goldberger's clinical electrocardiography: a Simplified Approach* (9th edn) (pp. 11–20). Philadelphia: Elsevier.)

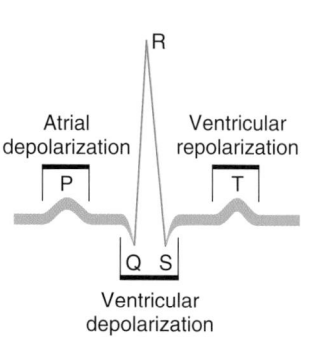

**Fig. 5.6** 'P' wave. (Little, J.W., Miller, C.S., Rhodus, N.L. (2018). Cardiac arrhythmias. In: *Little and Falace's dental management of the medically compromised patient* (9th edn) (pp. 70–85). St. Louis, MO: Elsevier.)

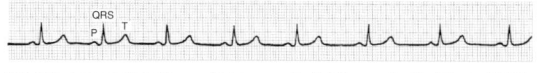

**Fig. 5.7** A normal ECG trace. (Goldberger, A., Goldberger, Z., Shvilkin, A. (2018). ECG basics: waves, intervals, and segments. In: *Goldberger's Clinical Electrocardiography: A Simplified Approach* (9th edn) (pp. 6–10). Philadelphia: Elsevier.)

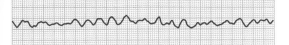

**Fig. 5.8** Ventricular fibrillation (lead II). (Hall, J., Hall, M. (2021). Cardiac arrhythmias and their electrocardiographic interpretation. *Guyton and Hall textbook of medical physiology* (14th edn) (pp. 157–168). Philadelphia: Elsevier.)

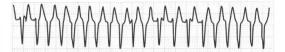

**Fig. 5.9** Ventricular tachycardia. (Schwartz, J., Lee, J., Hamrick, J., et al. (2017). Cardiopulmonary resuscitation. In: P. Davis, F. Cladis, *Smith's anesthesia for infants and children* (9th edn) (pp. 1236–1281). Philadelphia: Elsevier.)

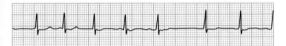

**Fig. 5.10** Atrial fibrillation. (Raftery, A., Lim, E., Östör, A. (2014). Palpitations. In: *Churchill's pocketbook of differential diagnosis* (4th edn) (pp. 370–372). Oxford: Elsevier.)

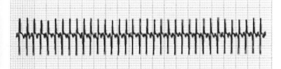

**Fig. 5.11** Supraventricular tachycardia. (Schwartz, J., Lee, J., Hamrick, J., et al. (2017). Cardiopulmonary resuscitation. In: P. Davis, F. Cladis, *Smith's anesthesia for infants and children* (9th edn) (pp. 1236–1281). Philadelphia: Elsevier.)

### Atrial fibrillation (Fig. 5.10)

Rate is variable but in the range of 150, there are no 'P' visible waves and there is an irregular rhythm.

### Supraventricular tachycardia (Fig. 5.11)

Rate in the range of 120, regular, QRS duration is normal, 'P' hard to distinguish as buried in the preceding 'T' wave.

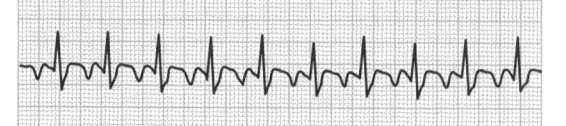

**Fig. 5.12** Atrial flutter. (Hall, J., Hall, M. (2021). Cardiac arrhythmias and their electrocardiographic interpretation. In: *Guyton and Hall textbook of medical physiology* (14th edn) (pp. 157–168). Philadelphia: Elsevier.)

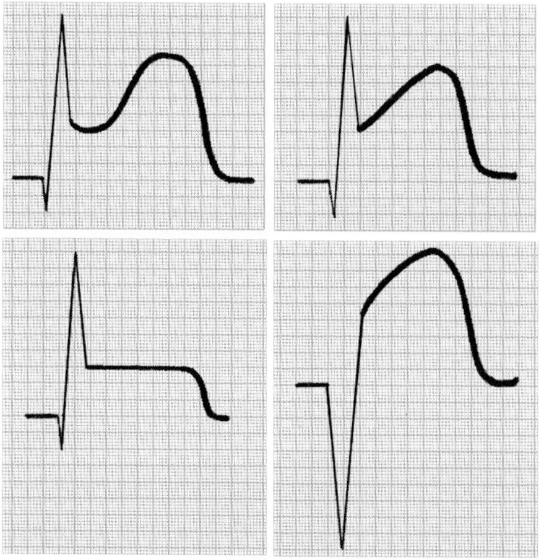

**Fig. 5.13** Variable shapes of ST segment elevations. (Goldberger, A., Goldberger, Z., Shvilkin, A. (2018). *Goldberger's clinical electrocardiography: a simplified approach* (9th edn) (pp. 73–91). Philadelphia: Elsevier.)

### Atrial flutter (Fig. 5.12)

Rate >150 bpm, rhythm regular, 'P' waves replaced with multiple flutter waves, usual at ratio of 2:1 or 3:1; that is, two flutter waves to one QRS.

### ST elevation (Fig. 5.13)

ST segment elevation of above 2 mm is not a normal finding on ECG and is indicative of ischaemic changes, which warrants urgent action.

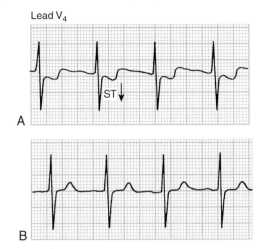

**Fig. 5.14** ST depression. **A,** Marked ST depressions seen in lead V4. **B,** Comparison normal ECG trace. (Goldberger, A., Goldberger, Z., Shvilkin, A. (2018). *Goldberger's Clinical Electrocardiography: A Simplified Approach* (9th edn) (pp. 92–103). Philadelphia: Elsevier.)

### ST depression (Fig. 5.14)

ST depression is also a potential sign of ischaemia and when seen in leads V1 to V4 is likely to indicate posterior myocardial infarct (MI).

### First-degree heart block (Fig. 5.15)

First-degree heart block is where the impulses conducted from the atria to the ventricles via the atrioventricular node are delayed to a period greater than 200 milliseconds.

### Second-degree heart block – Mobitz type I (Wenckebach) (Fig. 5.16)

A rhythm in which a progressive delay occurs in the conduction of electrical impulses through the AV node until conduction is completely blocked. The delay worsens with each P wave. The rhythm is characterized by progressive lengthening of the PR interval until a QRS complex fails to appear after the P wave.

- Rate is normal
- Rhythm is regularly irregular
- QRS duration is normal

### First-Degree AV Block

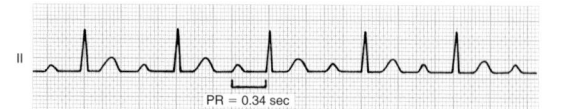

**Fig. 5.15** First-degree heart block – atrioventricular (AV) block. (Goldberger, A., Goldberger, Z., Shvilkin, A. (2018). Atrioventricular (AV) conduction abnormalities, part I: delays, blocks, and dissociation syndromes. In: *Goldberger's Clinical Electrocardiography: A Simplified Approach* (9th edn) (pp. 172–182). Philadelphia: Elsevier.)

### Mobitz Type I (Wenckebach) Second-Degree AV Block

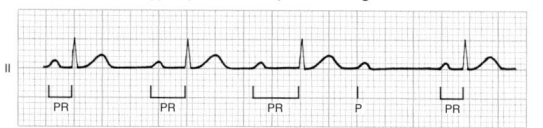

**Fig. 5.16** Second-degree heart block – Mobitz type I (Wenckebach). (Goldberger, A., Goldberger, Z., Shvilkin, A. (2018). Atrioventricular (AV) conduction abnormalities, part I: delays, blocks, and dissociation syndromes. In: *Goldberger's Clinical Electrocardiography: A Simplified Approach* (9th edn) (pp. 172–182). Philadelphia: Elsevier.)

### Mobitz II AV Block with Sinus Rhythm

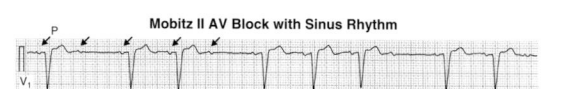

**Fig. 5.17** Second-degree heart block type – Mobitz type II. (Goldberger, A., Goldberger, Z., Shvilkin, A. (2018). Atrioventricular (AV) conduction abnormalities, part I: delays, blocks, and dissociation syndromes. In: *Goldberger's Clinical Electrocardiography: A Simplified Approach* (9th edn) (pp. 172–182). Philadelphia: Elsevier.)

- 'P' wave ratio 1:1 for 2, 3 or 4 cycles then 1:0
- 'P' wave rate is normal but faster than QRS rate

### Second-degree heart block – Mobitz type II (Fig. 5.17)

A rhythm characterized by intermittent, yet complete, block of electrical conduction below the AV node. This block occurs when a complete block of one bundle branch is accompanied by an intermittent block in the other bundle branch. This pattern produces an AV block characterized by absent (dropped) QRS complexes, usually

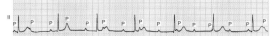

**Fig. 5.18** Third-degree heart block. (Goldberger, A., Goldberger, Z., Shvilkin, A. (2018). Atrioventricular (AV) conduction abnormalities, part I: delays, blocks, and dissociation syndromes. In: *Goldberger's Clinical Electrocardiography: A Simplified Approach* (9th edn) (pp. 172–182). Philadelphia: Elsevier.)

producing an AV conduction ratio of 4:3 or 3:2. Second-degree type II AV block is also referred to as Mobitz type II second-degree AV block.

- Rate is normal or slow
- Rhythm is regular
- QRS duration is prolonged
- 'P' wave ratio 2:1 or 3:1
- 'P' wave rate is normal but faster than QRS rate
- P–R rate is normal or prolonged but constant

### Third-degree heart block (Fig. 5.18)

This is a rhythm caused when the electrical impulse through the AV node, bundle of His, and bundle branches and characterized by 'P' wave and QRS complexes are completely dissociated (Wesley 2016).

### Heart auscultation locations (Fig. 5.19)

### Heart sounds

Auscultation findings fall into the following three categories:

- Heart sounds
- Murmurs
- Rubs

**Heart sounds** are brief, transient sounds produced by valve opening and closure; they are divided into systolic and diastolic sounds. On auscultation there are two sounds, the S1 and S2, which are followed by a short period of silence; these noises equate to muscular activity of the heart or the systolic phase of the cardiac cycle, whereas the short silence that follows is the diastolic phase, where the heart is at rest. Sounds heard between S1 and S2 are systolic sounds, and sounds heard between S2 and S1 are diastolic (Olson 2014).

**Murmurs** are produced by blood flow turbulence and are more prolonged than heart sounds; they may be systolic, diastolic or continuous. They are graded by intensity and are described by their location and when they occur within the cardiac cycle. Murmurs are graded in intensity on a scale of 1 to 6.

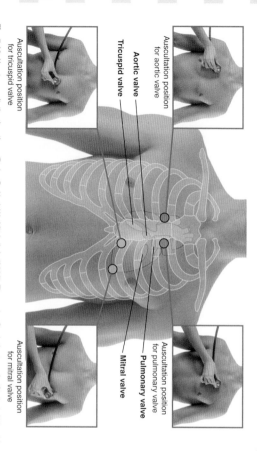

Auscultation position for aortic valve

**Aortic valve**

**Tricuspid valve**

Auscultation position for tricuspid valve

Auscultation position for pulmonary valve

**Pulmonary valve**

**Mitral valve**

Auscultation position for mitral valve

**Fig. 5.19** Heart auscultation locations. (Drake, R., Vogl, W., Mitchell, A. (2020). Thorax. In: *Gray's Anatomy for Students* (4th edn) (pp. 123–247). Philadelphia: Elsevier.)

**Rubs** are high-pitched, scratchy sounds often with two or three separate components; during tachycardia, the sound may be almost continuous.

The clinician focuses attention sequentially on each phase of the cardiac cycle, noting each heart sound and murmur. Intensity, pitch, duration and timing of the sounds and the intervals between them are analysed.

| | |
|---|---|
| **Mitral regurgitation** | The murmur of mitral regurgitation is mid-frequency, taking up all of systole with a third heart sound gallop in diastole. The murmur is caused by turbulent flow through the incompetent mitral valve leaflets into the left atrium. |
| **Aortic stenosis** | The murmur is loud and higher pitched and is caused by calcification of the aortic valve leaflets. There is a fourth heart sound, which is heard in late diastole (just before the first heart sound). An aortic ejection can be a click, heard in milder cases of aortic stenosis. |
| **Aortic regurgitation** | The first heart sound is diminished due to pre-mature closure of the mitral valve leaflets. An aortic ejection click follows the first heart sound. |
| **Mitral stenosis** | The first heart sound is increased in intensity while the second heart sound is normal. There is a low-pitched rumbling murmur that starts after the opening snap and lasts until mid-diastole. |
| **Ventricular septal defect** | The first heart sound is normal; there is, however, further turbulent flow into the left ventricle from the left atrium causing the diastolic murmur. This is caused by VSD-induced increased blood flow across the mitral valve. |

## References

Hampton, J. (2019). *The ECG made easy* (9th edn). London: Elsevier.

Olson, K., Rawlings, K. (2014). *Oxford handbook of cardiac nursing* (2nd edn). Oxford: Oxford University Press.

Wesley, K. (2016). *Huszar's ECG and 12-lead interpretation* (5th edn). London: Elsevier.

## Further Reading

O'Keefe, J.H., Hammill, S.C., Freed, M. *The complete guide to ECGs A comprehensive study guide to improve ECG interpretation.* Oxford: Blackwell.

Shea, M.J., Gupta, J.I. (2019). *Electrography.* MSD manual. Available at: https://www.msdma-nuals.com

# CHAPTER 6 Disability (Neurological System)

- Glasgow Coma Scale
- Acutely raised intracranial pressure (ICP)
- Meningitis
- Meningitis management
- Stroke management

Neurological assessment is a key skill of the nurse, as persevering neurological health could be considered as core to all healthcare, particularly in acute and deteriorating circumstance. The following are some key neurological assessment tools and guidance on some of the more commonly encountered neurological illnesses and situations (Simon et al 2017).

## Glasgow Coma Scale

### Glasgow Coma Scale (GCS)

| Eye opening (E) | Verbal response (V) | Motor response (M) |
|---|---|---|
| 4 = Spontaneous | 5 = Orientated | 6 = Obeys commands |
| 3 = To voice | 4 = Confused | 5 = Localize to pain |
| 2 = To pain | 3 = Incoherent words | 4 = Withdrawal from pain |
| 1 = None | 2 = Incomprehensible | 3 = Flexion to pain |
| | 1 = None | 2 = Extension to pain |
| | | 1 = None |

Total = E + V + M

Look for equal pupils with a brisk reaction to light (good tug).
Unequal pupils may be a sign of third cranial nerve palsy.
Raised blood pressure with bradycardia can indicate raised intracranial pressure.

## Raised intracranial pressure in the context of acute pathology or trauma

Acute raised intracranial pressure (ICP) constitutes a medical emergency as the nature of the non-compliant box of the skull does not allow for changes in pressure and volume of the brain, and tissues adjacent to the brain. Rapid onset of detrimental neurologic symptoms will follow if this situation remains unresolved. Raised ICP relative to oedema has three source mechanisms:

- Vasogenic – increased vaso-permeability due to tumour, trauma, ischaemia and infection
- Cytotoxic – cell death from hypoxia
- Interstitial – for example, obstructive hydrocephalus

## Causes

- Tumour
- Head injury

- Meningoencephalitis
- Brain abscess
- Hydrocephalus
- Cerebral oedema
- Haemorrhage – subdural, extradural, subarachnoid, intracerebral, intraventricular

## Raised ICP presentation

- Headache
- Drowsiness
- Vomiting
- Seizures
- Restlessness
- Reduced level of consciousness
- Irritability
- Falling pulse rate
- Raising B/P
- Coma
- Pupillary constriction, followed by later stage dilatation

## Management of raised ICP

- Use ABC approach to ensure appropriate prioritization and recognition of severity
- Treat hypotension associated with raised ICP
- Define cause
- Elevate bed head
- Intubate and ventilate in order to reduce $pCO_2$ thereby creating vasoconstriction, which is very effective at reducing ICP
- Osmotic agents, such as mannitol, are of some value
- Give dexamethasone
- Manage in ICU environment
- Treat cause

## Meningitis

Meningitis is an infection of the protective tissues, the meninges, that surround and protect the brain (Trunkel et al 2004).

Meningitis can be classified by duration or by aetiology:
- Duration: acute presentation within 24 hours of onset of symptoms; sub-acute, with symptoms lasting from 1–7 days; and chronic, with symptoms lasting more than 7 days.
- Aetiology: meningitis can by bacterial, viral or fungal.

Meningitis is a medical emergency, particularly meningococcal meningitis, which is a condition that is very rapidly progressive.

## Meningitis presentation

- Headache
- Neck stiffness
- Photophobia

- Positive Kernig's sign (pain and resistance on passive knee extension when hips are fully flexed)
- Non-blanching rash (roll a glass over the skin lesion, which remains in spite of the pressure)
- Possible seizures
- Nausea and vomiting

## Management

In the case of meningococcal meningitis, antibiotics should be commenced immediately, as this condition has a very high mortality rate.

When treating, consider most likely organism and select antibiotic accordingly:

- A common choice is benzylpenicillin and cefotaxime.
- Otherwise follow advice from microbiologist following return of culture and sensitivity from cerebral spinal fluid.

  Consider prophylaxis antibiotic therapy for any contacts.

  This organism is not aerosolized, and it is said kissing contact is the level of contact that puts individuals at risk.

  Isolate suspected bacterial meningitis. There is no need to isolate viral meningitis.

## Stroke

- Recent advance in stroke management and the inception of the stroke network have meant the rapid identification and diagnosis of stroke can enable the movement of the patient to a specialist centre where treatment can be carried out, which can have a massive positive effect on outcome.
- Sudden onset or deterioration over hours or days that occurs in step-by-step progression
- May have flaccid hemiplegia that becomes spastic
- May be unconscious
- May have dysphasia or aphasia
- Possible myriad of other focal and widespread neurological symptomology:

  Rapid assessment and diagnosis is essential.

  Confirmation of diagnosis is required and differentiation between a thrombus or bleed by CT scan.

  Treatment should begin within three hours of onset of symptoms.

  Management options are thrombolysis and thrombectomy.

  Contraindications to thrombolysis are recent infarct, any concurrent bleed and coagulopathy or anticoagulant therapy and recent surgery (Markus et al 2010).

## References

Markus, H., Pereira, A., Cloud, G. (2010). *Stroke medicine* (3rd edn). Oxford: Oxford University Press.

Simon, R.P., Greenberg, D., Aminoff, M.J. (2017). *Lange clinical neurology* (3rd edn). New York: McGraw-Hill Education/Medical.

Trunkel, A., Hartman, B.J., Kaplan, S.L., et al. (2004). Practice guidelines for management of bacterial meningitis. *Clinical Infectious Diseases*, 39(9), 1267–1284.

- Abdominal assessment
- Musculoskeletal assessment

In the ABCDE approach to patient examination the exposure of the patient will allow for further visualization and more in-depth examination of problems that the patient may be encountering. Here are some useful insights and approaches to some examination techniques (Walker et al 2017).

## The abdomen (Fig. 7.1)

### Abdominal examination

#### First glance assessment
- Does the patient look pale (bleeding)?
- Mottled (poor perfusion/dry)
- Yellow (jaundice)
- Alert and conversant
- Is the patient lying rigidly as though suffering with extreme pain?

#### History
- Location of pain
- Type of pain
- What relieves the pain?
- How long has it been a problem?
- Other symptoms such as nausea and vomiting
- Blood in vomit
- Blood in stools

#### Possible conditions
- Hernia – with acute pain, local discoloration, bloody stools, fever, fatigue; consider incarceration
- Appendicitis
- Pancreatitis
- Pelvic ulceration
- Inflammatory bowel syndrome (IBS)
- Pelvic inflammatory disease (PID)
- Bowel obstruction
- Renal calculi
- Distension
- Ascites
- Liver disease – spider nevi

#### On examination
- On palpation, does the pain worsen?
- Where is the pain located?

### Surgical emergencies: the acute abdomen

- Acute presentation
- Systemically unwell
- Signs and symptoms within the abdomen

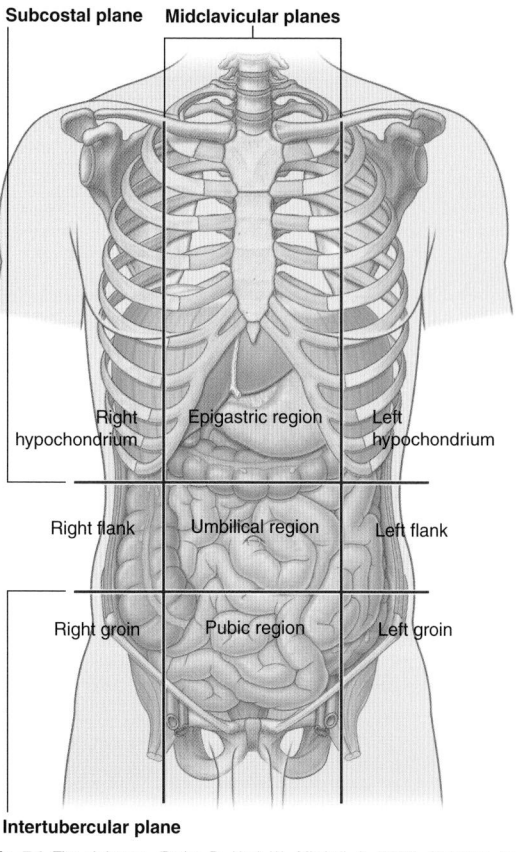

**Subcostal plane**  **Midclavicular planes**

Right
hypochondrium

Epigastric region

Left
hypochondrium

Right flank

Umbilical region

Left flank

Right groin

Pubic region

Left groin

**Intertubercular plane**

**Fig. 7.1** The abdomen. (Drake, R., Vogl, W., Mitchell, A. (2020). Abdomen. In: *Gray's Anatomy for Students* (4th edn) (pp. 249–412). Philadelphia: Elsevier.)

*Signs*
- Look for signs of shock
- Low blood pressure
- Postural drop in blood pressure
- Tachycardia

- Peripherally shut down
- Cap refill >2 seconds
- Look for signs of peritonitis, significant pain with board-like rigidity
- Shock
- Laying extremely still
- Abdominal pain on coughing
- Rebound tenderness
- Hyperactive or absent bowel sounds
- CXR may show sub-phrenic air if perforated bowel

### Possible cause
- Perforation of internal organs
- Rupture of appendix
- Infected peritoneal dialysis catheter in renal patients
- Following blunt trauma to abdomen

## Bowel obstruction

### Presentation
- Nausea and vomiting
- Colicky abdominal pain
- Distension
- Altered bowel habit; can be absolute constipation with no wind being passed
- High obstruction tinkling bowel sounds might be heard
- Bowel sounds may be absent

### Further investigations
- Abdominal X-ray, which may show excess gas in dilated hoop of gut
- Excess fluid levels on erect film

### Management
- If strangulated hernia, then urgent surgery needed
- Rupture of internal organ such as appendix will need surgery
- Otherwise pass nasogastric tube which is left on free drainage
- IVI hydration
- Nil by mouth
- Analgesia

(Heitkemper 2017)

## Musculoskeletal assessment

Musculoskeletal (MSK) assessment is a core element of nursing assessments and
what follows is a guide to some key areas in this field of practice (Egol et al 2014).

---

### MSK assessment approach

- Visualize
- Compare to other limb, if possible
- Palpate affected area, taking care in instances of suspected fracture not to
  move the fractured bone
- Look for loss of symmetry
- Note changes in gait

---

**MSK assessment approach—cont'd**

**Note:**
- Deformity
- Loss of motor function
- Pain and/or loss of sensation
- Localized oedema

## Management of fractures

- Visualize affected area
- Cover any wounds in instances of open fracture
- Immobilize affected limb
- Analgesia
- Manage shock
- Further care would be plaster of Paris or surgery
- Intravenous fluids
- Antibiotic therapy
- Analgesia

(Foster et al 2006)

**Fractured neck of femur.** This is a common injury in the elderly and is associated with a high mortality rate, with 10% of people with a hip fracture dying within a month of admission and 30% within 12 months. These deaths aren't all directly related to the fracture but rather reflect the high prevalence of comorbidity in people with hip fractures (NICE 2017).

### Presentation
- Typically history of a fall, but not always
- Leg shortening
- External rotation of affected limb
- Pain

### Management
- Prompt surgery within 48 hours if patient is fit for surgery
- Optimization pre-surgery, these patients may have been laying immobile at home for some time before being transferred to hospital – check bloods, particularly CK, as rhabdomyolysis is a high risk
- Effective analgesia before and after surgery
- Referral to orthogeriatrician on admission
- Early discharge to community-based rehabilitation
- Nerve block for pain is often used in management as effective analgesia helps with mobilization after surgery, which is crucial in this vulnerable patient group.

## GALS (Gait, Arms, Legs, Spine)

GALS examination is often used as a quick screening tool in musculoskeletal disorders to detect locomotor abnormalities and functional disabilities. This system was devised by Doherty et al (1992), who created this system as a quick, simple and sensitive system of screening for locomotor disorders.

The examination process involves observation, observation in motion, and palpation. The observation will identify deformity, asymmetry, reduced range of motion, stiffness, loss of muscle bulk, swelling, pain and pain on palpation.

## GALS Examination Record

|  | Appearance | Movement |
| --- | --- | --- |
| Gait | √ | √ |
| Arms | √ | X |
| Legs | √ | √ |
| Spine | √ | √ |

**Note:** Swollen wrist with reduced movement on the left side

The table above provides an example of how the GALS result will be displayed with a note of problems found, which may lead to further examination and testing/imaging (Foster et al 2006).

# References

Doherty, M., Dacre, J., Dieppe, P., Snaith, M. (1992). The 'GALS' locomotor screen. *Annals of the Rheumatic Diseases*, 51(10), 1165–1169.

Egol, K.A., Koval, K.J., Zuckerman, J.D. (2014). *Handbook of fractures* (5th edn). London: Wolters-Kluwer.

Foster, H.E., Kay, L.J., Friswell, M., et al. (2006). Musculoskeletal screening examination (GALS) for school aged children based on adult GALS screen. *Arthritis Care and Research*, 55(5), 709–716.

Heitkemper, M., Lewis, S., Dirksen, S., Bucher, L. (2017). *Medical surgical nursing: assessment and management of clinical problems*. London: Mosby.

National Institute for Health and Care Excellence (NICE). (2017). *Hip fracture: management* [CG124]. London: NICE. Available at: https://www.nice.org.uk/guidance/cg124

Walker, H.K., Hall, W.D., Hurst, J.W. (2017). *Clinical methods: the history, physical, and laboratory examinations* (3rd edn). Boston: Butterworth's.

# Further Reading

Baid, H'. (2009). A critical review of auscultating bowel sounds. *British Journal of Nursing*, 18(18), 1125–1129.

# CHAPTER 8 Resuscitation Council Algorithms for the Adult

- Achieving good outcomes
- Adult Basic Life Support
- Defibrillation algorithm
- Automated external defibrillation (AED) algorithm
- Using AED safely
- Cardiac arrest management
- Adult Advanced Life Support (ALS) algorithm
- Bradycardia/tachycardia algorithm
- Anaphylaxis

## Achieving good outcomes

A prompt and efficient cardiac arrest response is a key nursing skill. The nurse is invariably the first on scene, the first to recognize cardiac arrest, and the first to initiate the resuscitation process (RCUK 2021c).

Remember, good outcome of cardiac arrest is reliant on:

- Early recognition with minimal delay
- Prompt call for expert help and equipment, particularly a defibrillator
- Prompt and effective chest compression (CPR)
- Early defibrillation
- Good post-arrest care

The Resuscitation Council has graded various levels of cardiac response competencies into various different courses: Basic Life Support (BLS; Fig. 8.1), Immediate Life Support (ILS) and Advanced Life Support (ALS).

The interventions and manoeuvres discussed here will include all levels of competencies, however the approach to resuscitation for the nurse should be to have an understanding that the procedure is an incremental approach where each intervention leads into the next, and the level of training each team member has achieved should not preclude them from an understanding or gaining insight into the whole process.

## Cardiac arrest

There are two pathways in cardiac arrest management – shockable and non-shockable. However, there are three types of cardiac arrest:

- Ventricular fibrillation (VF) and pulseless ventricular tachycardia (VT), which are collectively known as shockable rhythms
- Pulseless electrical activity (PEA) – non-shockable rhythm
- Asystole – non-shockable rhythm

VF and pulseless VT are terminal rhythms in that, without intervention, they will result in death. It is essential, therefore, to have access to an AED and be able to deploy it effectively and safely (RCUK 2021b).

## Defibrillation (Fig. 8.2)

- Defibrillation works most effectively on oxygenated myocardium; therefore, good chest compressions with minimal interruptions are key

—√ 2021

**Adult basic life support in community settings**

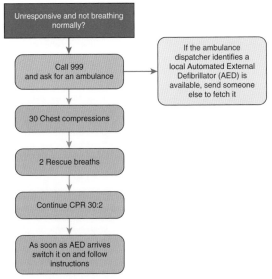

**Fig. 8.1** Adult Basic Life Support algorithm. (Resuscitation Council (UK). (2021). *Adult Basic Life Support* [online]. Available at: https://www.resus.org.uk/library/2021-resuscitation-guidelines/adult-basic-life-support-guidelines.)

- Shocks are given singularly every two minutes to enable myocardial oxygenation between each shock
- Biphasic defibrillation is preferable to monophasic

**Defibrillation and the automated external defibrillator (AED).** Electrical defibrillation is well established as the only effective therapy for cardiac arrest due to VF or pulseless VT.

Restoration of effective ventricular contraction is paramount in this situation, as cerebral hypoxic injury occurs after three minutes, less if there was a period of hypoxia prior to the arrest.

Defibrillation is the depolarization of a critical mass of myocardium simultaneously, to allow the restoration of the underlying natural pace-making function within the heart tissue.

**Chain of survival**

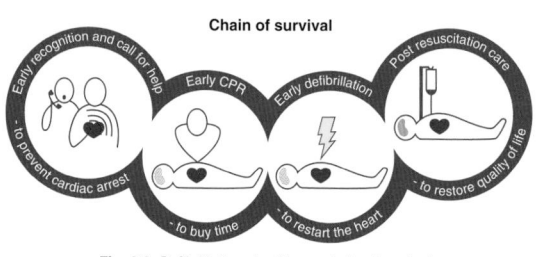

**Fig. 8.2** Defibrillation algorithm – chain of survival.

In many environments in and outside of the clinical settings, the automated external defibrillator (AED; Fig. 8.3) is the equipment of choice. The advantage of this equipment is:

- Ease of use, as there are verbal prompts throughout.
- Safety, as the AED is hands-free when the defibrillation shock is given.
- Biphasic waveform, which delivers lower energy to the myocardium thereby causing less damage. Biphasic defibrillation has a first shock efficacy of 90% and is significantly more successful than monophasic waveform defibrillation.

### Using an AED safely

The operator of the AED is responsible for the safety of all members of the team at the time of use.

- Assess the patient
- Apply pads
- AED will analyse; with the verbal prompt analysing, do not touch the patient
- When you are prompted 'shock advised'
- Ensure everybody is standing away from the patient
- Shout 'Oxygen away'
- State 'Charging stand clear'
- When charge available, shout 'Stand clear'
- Check everybody is clear
- Deliver shock

*Pad location.* The location of the pad is represented in diagram form on the pads themselves. The first location is the right side of the chest wall, just below the clavicle, with the second on the lower left side of the chest wall.

If the patient is wet due to sweat or some other body fluid, the skin should be dried to reduce the risk of arching electricity at the time of defibrillation.

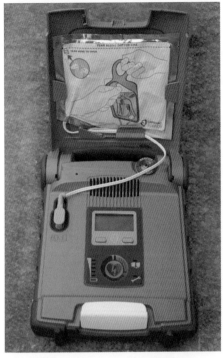

**Fig. 8.3** Automated external defibrillator (AED).

With the particularly hairy patient it can be useful to shave the area where the pads are to be placed to achieve better contact, however this should not delay defibrillation and most modern pads have heavy duty adhesive gel, making the likelihood of good contact high.

#### Cardiac arrest management

Good cardiac arrest management or indeed the management of any clinical emergency is most effective when there is:

- Good leadership
- Calm and clear communication
- Clear and agreed plan (the agreed ALS algorithm; Fig. 8.4)

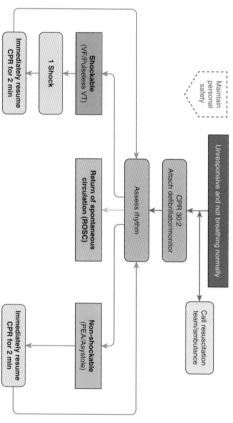

# Adult advanced life support

**Unresponsive and not breathing normally**

↓

Call resuscitation team/ambulance

↓

**CPR 30:2**
Attach defibrillator/monitor

↓

Assess rhythm

Maintain personal safety

**Shockable**
(VF/Pulseless VT)

→ 1 Shock → Immediately resume CPR for 2 min

**Return of spontaneous circulation (ROSC)**

**Non-shockable**
(PEA/Asystole)

→ Immediately resume CPR for 2 min

Resuscitation Council UK

GUIDELINES 2021

| Give high-quality chest compressions, and: | Identify and treat reversible causes | Consider | After ROSC |
|---|---|---|---|
| • Give oxygen<br>• Use waveform capnography<br>• Continuous compressions if advanced airway<br>• Minimise interruptions to compressions<br>• Intravenous or intraosseous access<br>• Give adrenaline every 3–5 min<br>• Give amiodarone after 3 shocks<br>• Identify and treat reversible causes | • Hypoxia<br>• Hypovolaemia<br>• Hypo-/hyperkalaemia/metabolic<br>• Hypo/hyperthermia<br>• Thrombosis – coronary or pulmonary<br>• Tension pneumothorax<br>• Tamponade – cardiac<br>• Toxins<br>Consider ultrasound imaging to identify reversible causes | • Coronary angiography/percutaneous coronary intervention<br>• Mechanical chest compressions to facilitate transfer/treatment<br>• Extracorporeal CPR | • Use an ABCDE approach<br>• Aim for SpO2 of 94–98% and normal PaCO2<br>• 12-lead ECG<br>• Identify and treat cause<br>• Targeted temperature management |

**Fig. 8.4** Adult Advanced Life Support algorithm. (Resuscitation Council (UK). (2021a). *Adult Advanced Life Support* [online]. Available at: https://www.resus.org.uk/library/2021-resuscitation-guidelines/adult-advanced-life-support-guidelines.)

- Leadership that is not compromised by being involved in tasks
- Stand at the foot of the bed so the whole resuscitation effort is easily visualized (Perkins et al. 2015)

The options in resuscitation are defibrillation for VF/VT or identify and manage the underlying cause in both PEA and asystole. All other manoeuvres are to support and optimize this management.

### Non-shockable pathway
- Chest compression CPR in two minutely intervals
- Give adrenaline 1 mg in 10 mL (1:10,000) 3–5 minute intervals
- Secure IV access
- Secure airway and give oxygen therapy
- Treat underlying cause

### VF/VT pathway (shockable pathway)
- Give single shocks of 150 joules biphasic or 360 joules monophasic
- Give single shock 2 minutely, resuming chest compression without delay as soon as administered
- Amiodarone 300 mg can be given after three unsuccessful shocks

## Reversible causes – the 4 Hs and the 4 Ts

### 4 Hs
- Hypoxia: secure airway and ensure good ventilation
- Hypovolaemia: secure access and give fluids and/or blood
- Hypo/hyperkalaemia/metabolic: potassium can be replaced if necessary; hyperkalaemia can be treated with sodium bicarbonate or calcium
- Metabolic causes include hypoglycaemia, for which glucose can be given
- Hypothermia: external warming device. Warm fluids into bodily cavities. Blood warmer infusion. Warming via dialysis.

### 4 Ts
- Thromboembolic–coronary or cardiac: thrombolysis and percutaneous coronary intervention, typically where arrest occurs in a cardiac catheter laboratory.
- Tension pneumothorax: decompression with a large-bore cannula in the second intercostal space mid-clavicular line.
- Cardiac Tamponade: decompression with needle pericardiocentesis. Normally determined by ultrasound.
- Therapeutic or toxic substance: possibilities are opiate and benzodiazepines; for opiate give naloxone initial 400 mcg IV with further doses dependent on response, and for benzodiazepines give flumazenil 200 mcg IV with 100 mcg doses following dependent on response.

## Drugs used in cardiac arrest

- Adrenaline 1 mg potentiates cerebral and cardiac tissue through a process of vasoconstriction, which increases perfusion pressure and can, it is thought, improve the outcome of the resuscitation but also, and crucially, preserve cerebral tissue.
- Atropine 3 mg is given to provide a blockade of the vagal nerve. This is a one-off 3 mg dose. Atropine should be given in asystole and in PEA when the monitored rhythm is bradycardia (below 60 bpm).

- Bicarbonate 50 mmol should be used to correct acidosis in or after the arrest situation where the arterial blood gas shows a pH of less than 7.1, or if the cardiac arrest is associated with tricyclic overdose or hyperkalaemia.
- Amiodarone 300 mg made up with 20% dextrose 20 mL given after three unsuccessful attempts at defibrillation. A further dose of 150 mg can be given for recurrent or refractory VF/VT, where no pre-filled syringes are available.
- Calcium chloride/calcium gluconate 10 mL of 10% can be given to treat hyperkalaemia, hypocalcaemia, calcium channel blocker overdose or an overdose of magnesium.

## Brady-/tachycardias

Bradycardia is a heart rhythm that is characterized by its slow rate, whereas tachycardia is a heart rate that is fast, when compared to normal heart rates at rest. The reason that these heart rates are important is that, at either a slow or fast rate, the heart can become incompetent in its function and not provide a sufficient pressure to perfuse the body organs, particularly cerebral tissue and the heart, which of course can have disastrous effect and cause serious illness and potentially death (Priori et al 2015).

These rhythms can in extremes put the patient into a peri-arrest situation and they consequently need prompt management.

**How the patient may appear:** pallor, sweaty, cold, clammy, peripherally shut down, impaired consciousness, confusion.

**Actions:** MOVE (see below); summon expert help.

### Move

**M** = Monitor: instigate cardiac monitoring. Observe all signs for further deterioration.

**O** = Oxygen is indicated in most peri-arrest situations. Administer high-flow oxygen. Caution should be taken in patients that are known to retain carbon dioxide.

**V** = Venous access: if the patient proceeds to cardiac arrest, establishing access ahead of time will be an invaluable intervention.

**E** = ECG & Expert help: an ECG is a useful intervention even if the problem is not cardiac-mediated, as other problems can be identified, such as electrolyte imbalance, for example.

### Tachycardia

In tachycardia the diastolic blood pressure is less well maintained, diastolic being the point at which coronary blood flow is achieved, therefore the patient is at high risk of myocardial ischaemia.

This phenomenon occurs at a different rate in broad complex tachycardia than in narrow complex tachycardia as the body tolerates broad complex tachycardia less well.

Risk of myocardial ischaemia occurs at rates of >200 beats per minute in narrow complex tachycardia, whereas in broad complex tachycardia the risk is significant at the lower rate of 150 beats per minute. See adult tachycardia (with pulse) algorithm (Fig. 8.5).

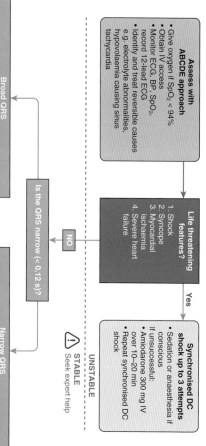

Resuscitation
Council UK

**Adult tachycardia**

**Assess with ABCDE approach**
- Give oxygen if SpO₂ < 94%
- Obtain IV access
- Monitor ECG, BP, SpO₂, record 12-lead ECG
- Identify and treat reversible causes e.g. electrolyte abnormalities, hypovolaemia causing sinus tachycardia

**Life threatening features?**
1. Shock
2. Syncope
3. Myocardial ischaemia
4. Severe heart failure

Yes

**Synchronised DC shock up to 3 attempts**
- Sedation or anaesthesia if conscious
- If unsuccessful: Amiodarone 300 mg IV over 10–20 min
- Repeat synchronised DC shock

**UNSTABLE**

NO

⚠ **STABLE**
Seek expert help

**Is the QRS narrow (< 0.12 s)?**

**Broad QRS**
Is QRS regular?

**Narrow QRS**
Is QRS regular?

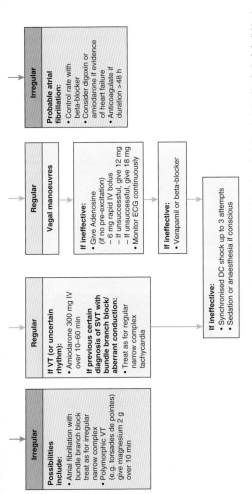

| Irregular | Regular | Regular | Regular | Irregular |
|---|---|---|---|---|
| **Possibilities include:** | **If VT (or uncertain rhythm):** | **Vagal manoeuvres** | | **Probable atrial fibrillation:** |
| • Atrial fibrillation with bundle branch block treat as for irregular narrow complex | • Amiodarone 300 mg IV over 10–60 min | | | • Control rate with beta-blocker |
| • Polymorphic VT (e.g. torsades de pointes) give magnesium 2 g over 10 min | **If previous certain diagnosis of SVT with bundle branch block/ aberrant conduction:** | **If ineffective:** | | • Consider digoxin or amiodarone if evidence of heart failure |
| | • Treat as for regular narrow complex tachycardia | • Give Adenosine (if no pre-excitation) | | • Anticoagulate if duration >48 h |
| | | – 6 mg rapid IV bolus | | |
| | | – If unsuccessful, give 12 mg | | |
| | | – If unsuccessful, give 18 mg | | |
| | | • Monitor ECG continuously | | |

**If ineffective:**
• Synchronised DC shock up to 3 attempts
• Sedation or anaesthesia if conscious

**If ineffective:**
• Verapamil or beta-blocker

Fig. 8.5 Adult tachycardia (with pulse) algorithm. (Resuscitation Council (UK). (2021). *Adult tachycardia (with pulse) algorithm* [online]. Available at: https://www.resus.org.uk/library/2021-resus citation-guidelines/adult-advanced-life-support-guidelines.)

59

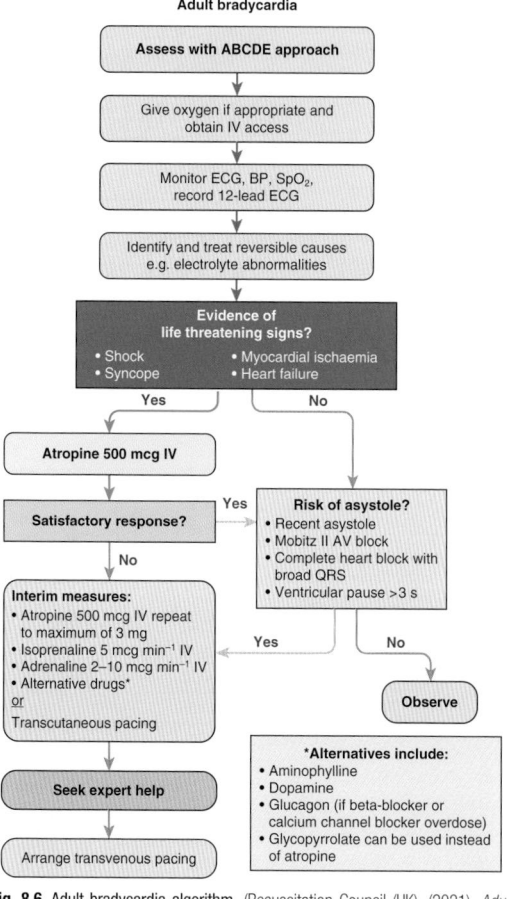

**Fig. 8.6** Adult bradycardia algorithm. (Resuscitation Council (UK). (2021). *Adult bradycardia algorithm* [online]. Available at: https://www.resus.org.uk/library/2021-resuscitation-guidelines/adult-advanced-lif e-support-guidelines.)

## Bradycardia

This is defined as less than 60 beats per minute, although a vulnerable patient with low cardiac reserve may well be symptomatic at a higher rate.

It should be noted that a bradycardia at this rate may be found in extremely fit patients, such as marathon runners, and does not need management and is in effect a normal finding in this patient group.

Similarly, treatment with beta blockers can induce a bradycardia without an insufficient cardiac output, therefore also likely to be non-problematic. See adult bradycardia algorithm (Fig. 8.6).

## Anaphylaxis

This is often a rapidly progressing and life-threatening condition, needing immediate action.

### Presentation

- Typically history of contact with allergen
- **Skin** changes with urticaria, and/or erythemic rash
- Itching, particularly close to the point of contact with allergen
- **Respiratory** changes with possible dyspnoea, wheeze, angioedema and stridor
- **Cardiovascular** changes, with hypotension, tachycardia, possible cardiac arrythmias and collapse
- Patient may well complain of a sense of impending doom, typically saying they feel as though they are going to die

### Action & treatment

- **Adrenaline** – repeat after 5 minutes if no significant improvement:
  - Adult and child above 12 years: 500 mcg IM
  - Child 6–12 years: 300 mcg IM
  - Child less than 6 years: 150 mcg IM
- **Chlorphenamine**
  - Adult and child above 12 years: 10 mg IV or IM
  - Child 6–12 years: 5 mg IV or IM
  - Child less than 6 years: 2.5 mg IV or IM
- **Hydrocortisone**
  - Adult and child above 12 years: 200 mg IV or IM
  - Child 6–12 years: 100 mg IV or IM
  - Child less than 6 years: 50 mg IV or IM
- **IV fluids N/saline**
  - Adult: 500–1000 mL
  - Child: 20 mL/L

In many organizations the adrenaline is available as an ampoule of 1 millilitre containing 1000 mcg, often described as 1 in 1000, and an amount needs to be drawn up to create the correct dosage; for example, in the adult in order to give 500 mcg, half a millilitre would need to be drawn up.

It should also be noted that the epipens that are prescribed to patients to use in an emergency, in the community do not have consistent dosages, although commonly in the adult they are 300 mcg (Simpson 2016).

## References

Perkins, G.D., Handley, A.J., Koster, R.W., et al. (2015). *ERC guidelines for Adult Basic Life Support and automated external defibrillation.* Brussels: European Resuscitation Council (ERC).

Priori, S.G., Blomstrom-Lundqvist, C., Mazzanti, A., et al. (2015). 2015 ESC Guidelines for the management of patients with ventricular arrhythmias and the prevention of sudden cardiac death: The Task Force for the Management of Patients with Ventricular Arrhythmias and the Prevention of Sudden Cardiac Death of the European Society of Cardiology (ESC). *European Heart Journal,* 36(41), 2793–2867.

Resuscitation Council (UK) (RCUK). (2021a). *Adult advanced life support guidelines.* London: Resuscitation Council (UK).

Resuscitation Council (UK) (RCUK). (2021b). *A guide to automated external defibrillators (AEDs).* London: Resuscitation Council (UK).

Resuscitation Council (UK) (RCUK). (2021c). *Resuscitation Council (UK) guidelines 2015.* London: Resuscitation Council (UK).

Simpson, E. (2016). In hospital resuscitation: recognising and responding to adults in cardiac arrest. *Nursing Standard,* 30(51), 50–63.

## Further Reading

National Institute for Health and Care Excellence (NICE). (2014). *Atrial fibrillation: the management of atrial fibrillation* [CG180]. London: NICE.

Nolan, J., Soar, J., Eikeland, H. (2006). The chain of survival. *Resuscitation,* 71(3), 270–271.

Soar, J., Nolan, J.P., Böttiger, B.W., et al. (2015). European Resuscitation Council Guidelines for Resuscitation 2015: Section 3. Adult advanced life support. *Resuscitation,* 95, 100–147.

## CHAPTER 9

Medical Emergencies

- Medical emergencies: the approach
- Myocardial infarction
- Acute asthma
- Gastrointestinal bleed (GIB)
- Hypoglycaemia
- Diabetic ketoacidosis
- Hyperglycaemic hyperosmolar non-ketotic coma (HONK)
- Status epilepticus
- Exacerbation of chronic obstructive pulmonary disease (COPD)
- Pulmonary oedema
- Acute kidney injury
- Hyperkalaemia
- Sepsis

When approaching the deteriorated patient, use the ABCDE approach to structure your initial assessment; the systematized approach allows a prioritization that facilitates the identification of the most urgent problems, in order that they can be found and dealt with promptly. The purpose of this process is to enable the rapid detection and resolution of the problem, and only after resolution can the assessment continue to the next stage (Wilson 2017).

A = Airway
B = Breathing
C = Circulation
D = Disability
E = Exposure
(See Ch. 2, General Assessment.)

Having undertaken this assessment, the nurse can move ahead to create a plan, which includes gaining further information, if necessary, and management of an appropriate action plan or algorithm, which are detailed here for some of the more compelling conditions.

## Management of acute myocardial infarct

### Presentation

- Pain, often central and crushing, can be severe retrosternal chest pain but can radiate to the arm, jaw, throat or shoulders. (Diabetic patients are sometimes known to present with no pain due to neuropathy. Often referred to as a silent myocardial infarct.)
- Typically nausea and vomiting
- May have tachy- or bradycardia depending on location of infarct
- Blood pressure may be high or low or even normal
- May be short of breath
- Feeling of impending doom

### Assessment

- ECG
- Enzymes

- Troponin T and troponin I
- Arterial blood gas (ABG)
- FBC, U&Es, LFTs, clotting studies

## Actions

- MOVE (monitor, oxygen, venous access, ECG and expert help)
- Serial ECG
- Analgesia: morphine 2.5–5 mg IV (this may need adjusting relative to patient size and renal function)
- Metroclopramide 10 mg
- Glycerol trinitrate infusion
- Intravenous beta-blocker
- Consider DVT prophylaxis
- Concurrent to all above: refer to cardiologist for percutaneous coronary intervention (PCI) or thrombolysis (NICE 2013b)

## Acute severe asthma

### Assessment

| Severe asthma | Life threatening asthma |
| --- | --- |
| Unable to complete sentences | Peak flow <33% of predicted best |
| Respiratory rate >25/minute | Silent chest |
| Pulse rate >110/minute | Cyanosis |
| Peak flow <50% of predicted best | Feeble respiratory effort |
| | Confusion |
| | Exhaustion |
| | Coma |
| | Bradycardia |
| | Arterial blood gases |
| | $pCO_2$ >5 kPa |
| | $pO_2$ <8 kPa |
| | pH <7.35 |

(HIS 2019)

## Actions

**M** – Monitor oxygen saturations, peak flow, and ABGs

**O** – Oxygen 100% via re-breath bag

**V** – Ensure venous access

**E** – Expert help of an anaesthetist or medical emergency team will most likely be needed

- Assess severity of attack
- Sit patient upright
- Salbutamol 5 mg nebulized with oxygen
- Hydrocortisone 200 mg I/V or 30 mg prednisolone
- CXR to exclude pneumothorax

If life-threatening:

- Ipratropium 0.5 mg with the nebulized salbutamol
- Aminophylline 5 mg per kg IV bolus over 20 minutes
- Consider salbutamol infusion
- Consider IV infusion of magnesium sulphate

If no improvement:

- Continue with 100% oxygen
- Nebulized salbutamol every 15 minutes
- Continue ipratropium 0.5 mg every 6 hours
- Consider ICU referral

## Gastrointestinal bleed

- Typical likely history of blood loss with vomit or in stool
- Likely shock, due to fall in circulating blood volume, secondary to blood loss and bleeding
- Potentially life-threatening

### Actions

- Managed ABC if reduced consciousness
- MOVE
- Insert two wide-bore cannula, one in each antecubital fossa
- Take bloods for cross-match, FBC and clotting studies + ABG (venous blood gas is also useful if the nurse in attendance is untrained in taking ABGs)
- Give large volumes of IV fluid
- If patient remains in shock, give O Rh-negative blood while awaiting cross-match

### Further actions

- Correct clotting abnormalities if found
- Secure central venous access
- Monitor fluid balance
- Arrange endoscopic investigation for diagnosis and management (Kumar & Clark 2016)

### Hypoglycaemia

#### Presentation

- Agitation
- Confusion
- Aggression
- Sweating
- Collapse

*In first aid scenario away from clinical environment, this presentation can be wrongly attributed to alcohol intoxication.

#### Actions

- Make diagnosis with blood glucose meter
- Ensure patient is not known to be an alcoholic or severely malnourished

- Secure IV access
- Give dextrose 50% in 50 mL (Caution with high-concentration dextrose, as the hyperosmotic nature of the fluid can cause vein damage and in extravasation can cause tissue damage; for this reason some organizations have only lower concentration available at 20%.)
- Repeat if no response after first dose
- If IV access is difficult to achieve, IM glucagon 1 mg, which should followed up with food to replenish stores of glycogen
- Follow up with diabetic referral or specialist diabetic nurse (Kumar & Clark 2016)

## Diabetic ketoacidosis

- This phenomenon can only occur with diabetes type 1
- Typically there is 2-to 3-day preamble with the following:
  - Polydipsia
  - Polyuria
  - Anorexia
  - Dehydration
  - Vomiting
  - Abdominal pain
  - Loss of appetite
  - Lethargy

Diagnosis is made in the presence of ketosis, acidosis with a pH of less than 7.3.

### Common preceding events

- Infection
- Recent surgery
- Myocardial infarction
- Wrongly prescribed insulin
- Non-complaint patient (commonly a patient suffering with anorexia nervosa)

### Management

- IV access with immediate infusion of large volume normal saline infusion
- Insulin 10 IU fast-acting if blood sugar >20 mmol/L
- Monitor potassium; serial ABGs will also enable surveillance of pH
- Give potassium (K+) replace titrated to serum K+
- Move on to sliding-scale insulin regime

## Hyperglycaemic hyperosmolar non-ketotic coma

- Affects non-insulin diabetics only
- Patients are invariably older
- Typically a week or so history of the presenting symptoms
- Polydipsia
- Polyuria
- Dehydration
- Vomiting
- Elevated blood glucose >35 mmol/L

- No ketones, as the patient has not switched to ketone metabolism
- Serum hyperosmolarity
- May present in a coma

## Management

- Rehydrate with large volumes of normal saline solution (Take care in the elderly with large-volume infusions.)
- Insulin in low dosages titrated to effect
- Monitor serum K+ and replace as necessary

## Status epilepticus

Status epilepticus is said to occur when a seizure lasts for more than 5 minutes or when recurrent seizures are so close together that the patient does not have time to recover in between.

### Actions

- Protect airway if necessary
- Protect patient from environment and self-injury
- Oxygen therapy 100% via re-breather mask
- IV access
- Test blood sugar
- Give dextrose 100 mL of 20% if indicated
- Take care if alcoholism suspected, and give thiamine 250 mg IV and Pabrinex ampoules 1 and 2 ahead of dextrose
- Observe closely

Usually after 5 minutes if seizure not terminated:

- Give lorazepam 4 mg slow IV bolus
- Or diazepam 10 mg PR if no IV access available
- If seizures continue, give phenytoin 15 mg/kg at a rate not exceeding 50 mg a minute with cardiac monitoring

If seizures continue beyond these interventions or if 30 minutes have elapsed before control is achieved, call for anaesthetic support.

## Chronic obstructive pulmonary disease (COPD) as acute presentation

An exacerbation of COPD can be infective or non-infective.

### Aim of treatment

- Manage hypoxia
- Manage asthmatic element of presentation
- Treat infection if present
- Refer back to long-term management

### Oxygen therapy starting with 24%

(Caution with $CO_2$-retentive patients, as lack of oxygen is often the stimulation to respiration in this chronic pathology, and radically increasing oxygen levels can have the effect of reducing respiratory rate and causing respiratory depression.)

With $CO_2$ retention it is appropriate to manage $O_2$ saturations to an agreed lower level, typically 88%–92%, or 92%–94% with oxygen therapy.

An ABG or VBG will guide the decision for which $O_2$ saturations to aim for.

## ABGs

Aim for $PaO_2$ >8.0 kPa
$PCO_2$ to fall by 1.5 kPa

## Further actions and treatment

- Nebulized salbutamol 5 mg 4-hourly or often back to back until symptoms resolving
- Ipratropium 0.5 mg 6-hourly
- IV hydrocortisone 200 mg and oral prednisolone 30 mg
- Auscultate and examine chest
- CXR
- Look for clinical signs of chest infection
- Rule out pneumothorax or pulmonary embolism as causation of acute presentation (There are well-established clinical prediction criteria for both, which are Wells score and PERC score, respectively.)
- Treat with antibiotics: amoxicillin 500 mg
- If pH <7.26 and $pCO_2$ is rising, refer on to a more intense environment or more aggressive management and support

## Intensives options

- **Non-invasive positive pressure ventilation (NIPPV)**
- **Intubation and ventilation:** if this option is being considered, it will be likely that the extremes of presentation are suggestive of a disease process that is very mature, therefore caution and due consideration should be given to the best interest of the patient. An insight into their pre-morbid functional status and life quality should be considered alongside comorbidities so that the best decision is made, as it is often difficult to wean patients from ventilation when they are suffering from COPD.
- **Respiratory stimulates such as doxapram:** less frequently used, this drug is considered a short-term adjunct while awaiting ventilation. Side effects: confusion, agitation, nausea and tachycardia.

## Pulmonary oedema

The causes of pulmonary oedema are varied but can often be related to cardiac disease or renal disease.

## Causes of pulmonary oedema

- Left ventricular heart failure following myocardial infarct or ischaemic heart disease
- Mitral valve stenosis
- Malignant hypertension
- Renal failure with fluid overload
- Inadequate dialysis and fluid control in the renal dialysis patient
- Acute respiratory distress syndrome (ARDS)

## Presentation

- The patent will feel distress and can describe a sense of impending doom
- Breathlessness
- Raised jugular venous pressure
- On chest auscultation, bilateral inspiratory crackles (see Ch. 4, Breathing (Respiratory Assessment)
- Hypertension
- Tachycardia
- CXR will show diffused white opacity with indistinct costophrenic margins, often with cardiomegaly

In ARDS, unless patient has ischaemic heart disease, the heart may appear normal in size.

## Management

- Nurse the patient in upright position
- MOVE
- Exercise caution when giving oxygen therapy to chronic $CO_2$-retaining patients such as COPD. If patient is hypercapnic (high $CO_2$) with a low to normal $HCO_3$ (bicarbonate), then it is likely to be acute and related to pulmonary oedema and therefore safe to give high-flow oxygen, ensuring close observation
- Diamorphine 2.5–5 mg
- Frusemide 40–80 mg
- Glyceryl trinitrate (GTN) two puffs or sub-lingual GTN 300 mg. Do not give in instance of hypotension where systole is below 90 mmHg
- Nitrate infusion if systole 100 mmHg or above, typical regime isosorbide dinitrate 2–8 mg IVI titrated against falling blood pressure
- If no or slow improvement, consider further frusemide 40–80 mg IV. Alternatively consider continuous positive airway pressure (CPAP) in place of incremental diuretic therapy

## Acute kidney injury (AKI)

Acute kidney injury (AKI), formerly acute renal failure, is where the kidney function declines in a sudden abrupt manner over a period of hours to days (Wilson 2017).

## AKI NICE criteria (NICE 2013a):

- Increase in serum creatinine 26 micromol/L or more within 48 hours
- 50% rise in creatinine occurring in the last seven days
- A fall in urine output to less than 0.5 mL/kg/hr for more than 6 hours

AKI and renal failure can arise in three different ways with three different mechanisms of causation. The first cause of renal failure is classified as prerenal, where the cause is not within the renal system but its effect is felt there, such as sudden acute loss of blood volume causing reduction in perfusion of the kidneys; this may happen with low blood pressure related to a major cardiac event, surgical blood loss, trauma, sepsis and myriad other causes. Intrinsic renal failure is where a problem arises within the kidneys and post-renal failure occurs when there is an issue preventing adequate draining of urine.

## Presentation

- Acute onset can be over hours or days
- Oliguria, anuria or polyuria depending on cause
- May have pulmonary oedema
- Systemic oedema may be present
- Bloods will show elevated urea creatinine and potentially potassium

## More common causes

- Acute tubular necrosis (ATN) most commonly associated with circulatory collapse
- Nephrotoxic agents such as:
  - NSAIDs
  - Aminoglycosides
  - Amphotericin B
  - Tetracyclines
  - ACE inhibitors
- Rhabdomyolysis
- Urinary tract obstruction
- Hepatorenal syndrome
- Sepsis

## Management

- MOVE
- Remove all previous access if sepsis is considered causative
- Monitor urine output – catheterize and measure output hourly
- Bloods:
  - U&Es
  - FBC
  - LFTs
  - Hepatitis serology
  - Autoantibodies
  - Blood cultures
- CXR for pulmonary oedema and cardiomegaly
- ECG – look for tall tented 'T' waves indicating high potassium
- Also observe for ectopic ventricular beats
- Renal tract ultrasound and KUB (kidney, ureter, bladder) imaging for obstructive cause
- Urine dipstick for protein and blood
- Urine microscopy:
  - White cell casts = possible infective cause
  - Red cell casts = possible inflammatory glomeruli cause
- Manage hyperkalaemia if present; dialysis may be indicated
- Fluid assessment: monitor urine output and observe for signs of fluid overload
- Treat oliguria if present with a low-volume intravenous fluid challenge:
  - 250–500 mL colloid or normal saline over 30 minutes
  - If fluid challenge is ineffective, repeat a second time
  - If elderly, low body mass or frail, take care with bolus volumes of fluid

- If oliguria persists:
  - Give frusemide with caution, as it can damage renal function
  - Renal dose dopamine 2–5 mcg per kilogram per minute
  - Manage acidosis with bicarbonate infusion: 50 mL of 8.4% sodium bicarbonate
  - Refer to renal physician if in fluid overload to pursue haemodialysis and/or haemofiltration

## Hyperkalaemia

Hyperkalaemia (elevated potassium) is a life-threatening condition which, if untreated, can lead to ventricular fibrillation (see Ch. 5, Circulation (Cardiovascular Assessment)). A potassium level of greater than 6.0 mmol/L will need emergency treatment.

However, there are instances when potassium of this level is routinely seen, for example in the chronic renal dialysis patient immediately prior to treatment.

### Some common causes

- Renal failure
- ACE inhibitors
- Potassium sparing diuretics
- Overdose of potassium supplements

### Management

- Nebulized salbutamol moves potassium from the extracellular space to the intracellular space
- Insulin and dextrose infusion
- 15–20 IU Actrapid insulin with 50% glucose
- Calcium gluconate 10 mL of 10% IV then calcium resonium 15 g three to four times a day
- Dialysis

## Sepsis

Sepsis is a profoundly significant problem with an estimated 37,000 deaths per year in England alone; these deaths are mostly preventable. The NHS launched an initiative in 2019 to improve the detection and management of sepsis and to raise awareness of the prevalence and urgency of this condition.

### Risk factors

- History of recent surgery, trauma, wounds and, in the elderly, pressure ulcers can be a source
- Impaired immunity, such as diabetes mellitus, renal failure and use of steroids, etc
- The very young
- The vulnerable, such as the elderly
- Indwelling catheters and other lines, e.g. central lines, cannulas

### Presentation and risk

- Altered mental state – confusion
- Reduced or impaired consciousness – GCS 14 or below

- Tachycardia of greater than 130 beats/min
- Hypotension with a systolic lower than 90 mmHg and/or a diastolic lower than 40 mmHg mercury
- Oliguria or anuria
- Mottled or ashen appearance
- Cyanosis

## Actions

- Manage ABCs if necessary
- Arterial blood gas (ABG) for lactate and glucose
- Blood cultures
- FBC, CRP and renal profile
- Give IV antibiotics within 1 hour of diagnosis
- Consider ICU/medical emergency team referral

## References

Healthcare Improvement Scotland (HIS). (2019). *SIGN 158: British guideline on the management of asthma.* Edinburgh: SIGN.

Kumar, P., Clark, M. (2016). *Clinical medicine* (9th edn). London: Elsevier.

National Institute for Health and Care Excellence (NICE). (2013a). *Acute kidney injury* [CG169]. London: NICE.

National Institute for Health and Care Excellence (NICE). (2013b). *Myocardial infarction with ST-segment elevation: acute management* [CG167]. London: NICE.

Wilson, I.B., Raine, T., Wiles, K., et al. (2017). *Oxford handbook of clinical medicine.* Oxford: Oxford University Press.

## Further Reading

Tintinalli, J.E., Stapczynski, S., Ma, O.J., et al. (2016). *Tintinalli's emergency medicine: a comprehensive study guide* (8th edn). New York: McGraw-Hill.

- Preoperative care and safety
- Postoperative care
- Postoperative nausea and vomiting (PONV)

In surgical care there are many considerations before and after the procedure that is performed in theatre; the following are some key issues for consideration and guidance for the nurse practising in this area (Lewis et al 2017).

### Safety and the WHO checklist (Fig. 10.1)

### Preoperative care

- In preparation for surgery the first priority is safety (Mehta et al 2006)
- Ensure the right person is having the correct surgery. Ensure the patient's identity is correct using at least three data points: name, DOB, hospital number
- Ensure correct procedure is scheduled
- Through the process of clerking and preoperative nursing assessment, ensure that the procedure planned is still appropriate
- Consider disease progression and determine whether relevance or efficacy of procedure is still current and still delivers benefit, and whether other options are now available
- Optimize patient prior to surgery: appropriate hydration, supplemented nutrition if possible, and offset any other known risk or problem as much as possible
- Achieve informed consent from the patient, ensure the patient understands the procedure planned and that the risk has been described and quantified

### Preoperative clerking and nursing assessment

Many nurses working in surgical specialties in practitioner roles will be responsible for clerking the patients. Here follows a clerking checklist:
- History of present complaint
- Past medical history
- Known allergies
- Current medication
- Social history
- Examination pertinent to the problem
- Note site for surgery and mark body if appropriate

It is often valuable to draw a picture of the lesions or morbid changes to an organ's structures relative to the presenting illness as an accurate record at a specific point in time; photography is also equally valuable, if available (Lewis et al 2017).

### Systemic exam

- Cardiovascular: ECG if over 60
- Respiratory exam assessing for any issues that might be a risk factor for an-aesthesia, such as long-standing respiratory disease or current chest infection
- Neurological base line
- Renal system with bloods to supplement findings

# WHO Surgical Safety Checklist
(adapted for England and Wales)

## SIGN IN (To be read out loud)

**Before induction of anaesthesia**

**Has the patient confirmed his/her identity, site, procedure and consent?**
- ☐ Yes

**Is the surgical site marked?**
- ☐ Yes/not applicable

**Is the anaesthesia machine and medication check complete?**
- ☐ Yes

**Does the patient have a: Known allergy?**
- ☐ No
- ☐ Yes

**Difficult airway/aspiration risk?**
- ☐ No
- ☐ Yes, and equipment/assistance available

**Risk of >500ml blood loss (7ml/kg in children)?**
- ☐ No
- ☐ Yes, and adequate IV access/fluids planned

## TIME OUT (To be read out loud)

**Before start of surgical intervention**
for example, skin incision

**Have all team members introduced themselves by name and role?**
- ☐ Yes

**Surgeon, Anaesthetist and Registered Practitioner verbally confirm:**
- ☐ What is the patient's name?
- ☐ What procedure, site and position are planned?

**Anticipated critical events**

**Surgeon:**
- ☐ How much blood loss is anticipated?
- ☐ Are there any specific equipment requirements or special investigations?
- ☐ Are there any critical or unexpected steps you want the team to know about?

**Anaesthetist:**
- ☐ Are there any patient specific concerns?
- ☐ What is the patient's ASA grade?
- ☐ What monitoring equipment and other specific levels of support are required, for example blood?

## SIGN OUT (To be read out loud)

**Before any member of the team leaves the operating room**

**Registered Practitioner verbally confirms with the team:**
- ☐ Has the name of the procedure been recorded?
- ☐ Has it been confirmed that instruments, swabs and sharps counts are complete (or not applicable)?
- ☐ Have the specimens been labelled (including patient name)?
- ☐ Have any equipment problems been identified that need to be addressed?

**Surgeon, Anaesthetist and Registered Practitioner:**
- ☐ What are the key concerns for recovery and management of this patient?

Name:
Signature of
Registered Practitioner

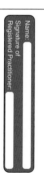

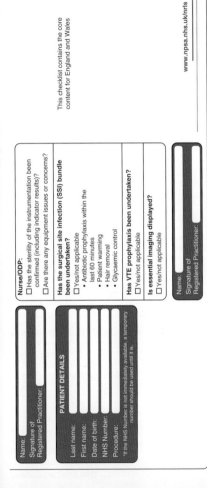

Name:
Signature of
Registered Practitioner:

**PATIENT DETAILS**

Last name:

First name:

Date of birth:

NHS Number:

Procedure:

*If the NHS Number is not immediately available, a temporary number should be used until it is.

**Nurse/ODP:**

☐ Has the sterility of the instrumentation been confirmed (including indicator results)?

☐ Are there any equipment issues or concerns?

**Has the surgical site infection (SSI) bundle been undertaken?**

☐ Yes/not applicable
  • Antibiotic prophylaxis within the last 60 minutes
  • Patient warming
  • Hair removal
  • Glycaemic control

**Has VTE prophylaxis been undertaken?**

☐ Yes/not applicable

**Is essential imaging displayed?**

☐ Yes/not applicable

This checklist contains the core content for England and Wales

Name:
Signature of
Registered Practitioner:

www.npsa.nhs.uk/nrls

**Fig. 10.1** WHO Surgical Safety Checklist (adapted for England and Wales). (Burbos, N., Morris, E. (2011). Applying the World Health Organization Surgical Safety Checklist to obstetrics and gynaecology. *Obstetrics, Gynaecology & Reproductive Medicine*, 21(1), 24–26).

## Preoperative blood tests

These blood tests are to identify problems that may be unknown or to quantify issues identified and, in the absence of illness, to create a base line:

- U&Es
- FBC
- Group and save and/or cross-match, depending on type of surgery
- Clotting studies
- Blood glucose
- LFTs
- C-relative protein (CRP) to rule out any unknown illness/infection that may predispose to greater risk

### Other tests

- ECG if over 60
- Chest X-ray if over 60 or known to present some level of respiratory risk

## Diabetic patients

- Ensure blood glucose is known
- Achieve control preoperatively using dextrous and insulin infusion (sliding scale)

## Postoperative management

- Postoperative management has five prime concerns: observation for systemic shock, observation for bleeding from site of surgery, fluid management, pain management and prevention/surveillance of infection
- Ensure regular vital sign recording, including B/P, pulse, temperature, respiratory rate, oxygenation
- Keep a fluid balance chart
- Record blood lost from wound and wound drains
- Visualize wound and/or dressing for signs of haemorrhage

## Hypotension and shock

There are four types of shock:

- Hypovolaemic, where there is insufficient circulating fluid volume
- Cardiac, where a problem intrinsic to heart function is making the blood ejected on each heartbeat less than needed, thereby creating low pressure
- Distributive, where the small blood vessels, through a pathological process, allow blood to pool peripherally, for example sepsis or anaphylaxis
- Obstructive shock, where the heart function is compromised by some local physical pathology, such as tamponade or pulmonary emboli

Postoperatively, hypotension is likely to be related to either the effects of the anaesthesia or hypovolaemic shock due to low volume (Mehta et al 2006).

### Management

- Tilt head of bed down
- Give oxygen
- Ensure large bore cannula
- Give fluids, N/saline or blood if haemorrhage is the cause
- Cardiac monitor if severe
- Consider intensivist support

## Postoperative temperature

- Pyrexia postoperatively in the first 24 hours is not uncommon and often relates to suboptimal ventilation of lungs at time of surgery
- Treat with physiotherapy and early mobilization
- Pyrexia beyond 24 hours or high temperature should prompt infection screen
- Examine chest
- Examine wound site
- Look for signs of pertonitis in abdominal surgery
- Urinary tract infection (UTI) particularity if catheterization has been undertaken
- Look for signs of DVT
- Send blood culture

## Shortness of breath post surgery

- Sit up
- Give oxygen therapy (caution $CO_2$ retentive)
- ABGs
- CXR
- Look for signs of pulmonary oedema
- Look for signs of pneumothorax
- Look for signs of atelectasis
- Treat findings

## Has not passed urine (HNPU)

- Common problem related to anaesthetic
- Encourage patient to stand if possible
- Walk to toilet if possible
- Stand patient close to running water, which can sometimes help
- Examine patient for palpable bladder
- Avoid catheterization unless absolutely necessary
- Undertake fluid assessment
- Ensure fluid replacement regime is correctly calculated

## Postoperative nausea and vomiting (PONV)

Nausea and vomiting are common problems in surgical procedures, particularly following anesthetic, and can cause many problems from increased postoperative pain and dehiscence of the surgical wound to electrolyte imbalance, dehydration and aspiration. Ideally this risk is managed with prophylactic anti-emetic therapy; however, this is not always effective, and treatment may have to be supplemented postoperatively.

### Action plan of management

- Identify cause
- Assess and manage hydration and perfusion problems related to hypovolaemia
- Consider and examine for paralytic ileus: use nasogastric drainage if necessary
- Review analgesia, as may be inadequate
- Review for signs of infection
- Visualize wound
- Consider if hypoxic: identify cause, give or supplement oxygen therapy, if appropriate
- Has appropriate or enough anti-emetic been given? Does it need supplementing?

**Common postoperative anti-emetics**

- Ondansetron 4 mg orally/IV every 8 hours
- Prochlorperazine 3–6 mg every 12 hours or 12.5 mg deep IM injection
- Droperidol (doses vary – see BNF for guidance)
- Cyclizine 50 mg oral/IM/IV every 8 hours

(See BNF for specific guidance.)

**Pain management postoperatively**

*Epidural.* Epidural administration of analgesia is an effective way of managing pain, where typically local anaesthetic and analgesia are infused into the epidural space (Malek et al 2017).

- Problems
- Respiratory depression
- Systemic effect on cardiovascular system can cause hypotension
- Loss of bladder control
- Headache
- Nausea

It is therefore particularly important to maintain close observation with a focus on respiratory function and blood pressure recordings.

*Patient-controlled analgesia (PCA).* This system has analgesia in an infusion where intermittent self-administered boluses can be delivered as necessary; the obvious benefit is that there is no wait for pain relief.

PCA has been a feature of postoperative pain control for some time and delivers further benefits over the intramuscular injection of analgesia; these include improved pain relief, greater patient satisfaction, lesser sedation and fewer postoperative complications.

## References

Lewis, S., Bucher, L., Heitkemper, M., et al. (2017). *Medical and surgical nursing: assessment and management of clinical problems* (10th edn). London: Elsevier.

Mehta, S., Hinmarsh, A., Rees, L. (2006). *Handbook of general surgical emergencies.* Oxford: Rafcliffe Publishing.

Malek, J., Ševčik, P., Bejšovec, D., et al. (2017). *Postoperative pain management* (3rd edn). Prague: Malada Vodami.

# Positive-Pressure Ventilation (NIPPV)

- Continuous positive airway pressure (CPAP)
- Biphasic positive airway pressure (BiPAP)
- Complications and nursing care

Non-invasive positive-pressure ventilation (NIPPV) is an intervention that provides respiratory support and has several different applications. The system consists of a well-fitting face mask and a closed circuit with an oxygen-enriched air supply, which is delivered in such a way as to create a positive expiratory end pressure.

The positive pressure in the breathing circuit ensures that the patient breathes against a resistance, which provides a number of benefits: it reduces the workload of breathing, improves ventilation and improves oxygenation.

There are two types of NIPPV, the first is continuous positive airway pressure (CPAP), and the second in biphasic positive airway pressure (BiPAP) (Sawkins 2001).

## Continuous positive airway pressure (CPAP)

CPAP has three applications:
- The first is in the management of type 1 respiratory failure, where there is a $PaO_2$ less than 8 kPa with a normal or low $PaCO_2$; in these circumstances the improvement of oxygenation is its prime purpose.
- The second use is in heart failure with associated pulmonary congestion, where the positive pressure applied in the respiratory cycle increases intrathoracic pressure, which in turn reduces both preload and afterload, reducing the workload of the heart. The positive pressure also works locally on the alveoli of the lung, pushing fluid back into pulmonary vasculature.
- The third use is in sleep apnoea, where the soft tissue collapses into the airway causing partial obstruction during sleep; with the use of CPAP the positive pressure acts directly on this soft tissue, reducing this partial obstruction and thereby enabling uninterrupted sleep.

## Biphasic positive airway pressure (BiPAP)

BiPAP delivers intermittent positive pressure at inspiration, which assists ventilation reducing $CO_2$ levels, and the lower pressure during the expiratory part of the breathing cycle enables greater oxygenation. BiPAP is therefore the choice of NIPPV treatment for type 2 respiratory failure where there is reduced $PaO_2$ and an increased $pCO_2$.

BiPAP is a valuable intervention particularly in the vulnerable patient group suffering with type 2 respiratory failure; as the disease process progresses, it can be increasingly difficult to wean these patients from ventilation, and BiPAP provides an alternative. BiPAP also uses less resource than ventilation, as it does not necessitate an intensivist environment.

## Complications and nursing care

Pressure sores to the nose bridge are a potential complication of this treatment, as the system is only effective if the mask fits tightly with no air leak, and consequently the mask is applied very tightly. There are dressings that can be used to protect the nose, such as hydrocolloid dressing, which can be used proactively to protect the nose bridge, and intermittent relief of pressure by lifting the mask away from the face is a useful intervention. When undertaking this care, it must be done in concert with the respiratory needs.

Claustrophobia and anxiety are also a common problem, and patients need to be reassured and comforted as much as possible. Any concern about suffocation can be offset by encouraging the patient to engage with the therapy, which in fact aids breathing. It is important to ensure that the patient has the call bell within easy reach so that they feel in control and can call for help if needed, although these patients should be in an environment of higher observation.

Patients can also find the positive pressure blows air into their eyes, which is uncomfortable and is also an indication of a poorly fitted mask.

With NIPPV the reduction in cardiac preload can cause a significant hypotension if the patient is hypovolaemic, so it is important to carry out a fluid assessment and ensure the patient is appropriately hydrated throughout treatment. In the acute setting this will necessitate intravenous fluid management and the use of a urinary catheter to accurately measure fluid balance (Wallis et al 2011).

## References

Healthcare Improvement Scotland (HIS). (2019). *SIGN 158: British guideline on the management of asthma*. Edinburgh: HIS/SIGN.

Sawkins, D. (2001). Non-invasive positive pressure ventilation. *Nursing Times*, 97(26), 52.

Wallis, C., Patton, J.Y., Beaton, S., Jardine, E. (2011) Children on long term ventilatory support: 10 years of progress. *Archives of Disease in Children*, 96(1), 998–1002.

## Further Reading

Tintinalli, J.E., Stapczynski, S., Ma, O.J., et al. (2016). *Tintinalli's emergency medicine: a comprehensive study guide* (8th edn). New York: McGraw-Hill.

- Cannulation
- Venepuncture

Accessing and managing the intravenous route is key in many areas of healthcare and a core skill for the nurse in practice (Barton et al 2017).

## Cannulation

Cannulation is a fundamental skill, whether in an emergency context of rapid vascular access being vital to advanced resuscitation manoeuvres, or as a prerequisite to the administration of key therapeutic intravenous agents.

### Before the procedure

- Identify the patient
- Ensure rationale is still current; for example, should this patient still be taking antibiotics intravenously, or is intravenous hydration still necessary?
- Gain informed consent
  ### *Considerations before undertaking the procedure*
- Patient's general circumstances: are there mental health or neurological problems?
- Allergies to latex plaster or tape
- Fears and phobias
- Faints
- Clotting disorders and possible use of anticoagulants

### The equipment

- 5-mL syringe
- Choice of cannula
- Gloves – the correct size is important, as palpating a vein though gloves that are too large can make the task near impossible
- Tourniquet
- Alcohol or chlorhexidine spray
- Cotton wool ball or gauze and tape
- Appropriate cannula dressing
- Sharps bin
- Choice of cannula
  - Size 14–16g in hypovolaemia
  - Size 18g for blood transfusion
  - Size 20–22g in all other cases
  - The smaller the cannula gauge size, the wider the bore of the cannula

### Selecting the vein

- Vein selection is the most important part of the procedure
- Ensure both you and the patient are comfortable, raise the bed or chair so you are at the correct height and do not have to bend
- Support the patients arm with a pillow or something similar

- Explain to the patient that an examination precedes the cannulation and that you will warn them immediately before the cannula is inserted
- Choose a site lower down the arm, unless the patient is likely to need aggressive fluid infusion, in peri-arrest or in cardiac arrest, in which case the antecubital fossa is more appropriate
- Palpate the vein to ensure it is elastic, which is often described as bouncy
- Note the path the vein takes
- Note the bends and change in direction of the vein

## What to avoid

- Fibrosed veins, which may appear in a good place to site a cannula but on palpation are hard to the touch and inelastic
- Inflamed veins
- Close to infection
- Bruising
- Directly over joints
- Side of cerebrovascular accident (CVA) or post-mastectomy
- Arm with infusion
- Dominant arm, if possible
- Avoid placing in the patient's hand unless no other vein is available, as this position is very uncomfortable for the patient and extravasates easily due to the frequent movement of the patient's hand

## Cannulation – the procedure

- Apply the tourniquet
- Don gloves (some clinicians will claim better success without gloves, as palpation is easier; this is a dangerous practice that should be discouraged)
- Clean skin and wait*
- Stretch the skin with your thumb underneath the insertion site to stabilize the vein
- Insert the cannula at 30 degrees. Use a slow and smooth action when inserting.
- Obtain a flashback. This is the movement of blood into the cannula port which tells you when you have breached the vessel wall with the metal tip of the inner steel tube that runs down the middle of the cannula.
- The polyurethane plastic catheter of the cannula is at this stage outside the vein as the steel protrudes beyond the catheter by a few millimetres
- At this point stabilize the cannula
- Advance the whole catheter a few millimetres
- Now advance the cannula catheter along the inner steel. The steel remains while this happens.
- It is at this point that most failed cannulations occur, as the inexperienced nurse will advance the catheter too early and it will buckle against the vessel wall*

---

*The correct use of alcohol wipes is dependent on the nurse vigorously wiping the area for a minimum of 1 minute and then allowing the area to dry for a further whole minute. In practice this does not always happen, and the practice of 'a quick wipe' can serve to agitate surface bacteria and in fact heighten the risk of infection being introduced at the time of cannulation.

### *Once cannula is in place*

- Release the tourniquet
- Remove the needle whilst compressing the vein with the thumb of your other hand
- Dispose of the sharp immediately (always have a sharps box beside you, placed before the procedure is undertaken)
- Attach a three-way tap extension primed with normal saline, to cap off
- Flush and confirm dressing
- Dispose of contaminants
- Complete insertion time and date sticker and affix at site
- Document using stickers from cannula pack

## Cannulation hints and tips to overcome difficulties

- Difficulty can occur in obesity, dehydration, the elderly, peripherally shut down and those with peripheral oedema
- Ensure tourniquet is applied tightly
- Put tourniquet on before preparing equipment, as it will allow greater time for the veins to fill
- Tapping veins can help but can be uncomfortable, so undertake with caution. Avoid before phlebotomy, as trauma to tissue can cause intracellular potassium to be released, erroneously affecting levels in blood sample
- Clenching and unclenching the fist can make the vein more available for cannulation
- A warm water dip can also make the veins expand

## Cannulation complications

- Infection localized to insertion site
- Systemic infection, as septicaemia can result from local infection
- Extravasation is a common complication of intravenous therapy, and in extreme cases, particularly where hypertonic solutions are used, it can lead to tissue damage up to and including necrosis
- Haematoma is also a common problem, and usually occurs at the time of insertion and is often related to poor technique at the time of advancing the cannula catheter
- Arterial puncture can occur if an unusual site is being used in the difficult-to-cannulize patient; when this occurs, strong and sustained pressure needs to be applied to the puncture site
- Once cannula is in use, a common complication is phlebitis; a useful way of observing the site, assessing the likelihood and/or severity of phlebitis, is the Visual Infusion Phlebitis Score, which will guide both assessment process and advice on best action (Phillips 2017).

## Venepuncture

Venepuncture is a skill that has become increasingly included as part of the nurse's role, and it should be considered as a skill that underpins and enables more advanced assessment and clinical management. The taking of blood should not be considered a stand-alone task where the nurse has no specific investment or indeed rationale with regard to the result of the ordered blood tests.

## Venepuncture – the procedure

- Apply the tourniquet
- Don gloves
- Have the correct and correctly labelled bottles
- Stretch the skin with your thumb underneath the insertion site to stabilize the vein
- Clean and wait. (Refer to cannulation section for further information on skin cleaning)
- Insert butterfly or needle bevel up at an angle of 30 degrees using a slow and smooth action of insertion.
- Obtain flashback. The butterfly has an advantage over fixed needle systems, as the difficult and small veins can be found more readily with a butterfly and there is no vacuum to collapse the smaller, more delicate veins. (Refer to the cannulation section for further information on vein selection and palpation.)

## Venepuncture with the vacutainer system

The vacutainer system has been designed to reduce the risk of infected needlestick injuries, by having an enclosed blood-filling system where the blood bottles are pre-charged with a vacuum. When this system is used correctly, the needle is only exposed at point of contact with the patient's skin, after which it is retracted into a closed and sealed compartment in the equipment. However, this system is available to misuse, and there are times when clinicians will draw blood with a conventional syringe and needle and then fill the bottles by manually puncturing them; this of course is a dangerous practice, as it means a potentially infected needle point is being directed at a blood bottle that is in the clinician's hand, making contact much more likely (Phillips et al 2017).

## References

Barton, A., Ventura, R., Vavrik, B. (2017). Peripheral intravenous cannulation: protecting patients and nurse. *British Journal of Nursing*, 26(8), S28–S33.

Phillips, S., Collins, M., Dougherty, L. (2011). *Venepuncture and cannulation*. Chichester: Wiley Blackwell.

## Further Reading

Dougherty, L., Lister, S. (1991). *The Royal Marsden manual of clinical nursing procedures* (9th edn). Chichester: Wiley Blackwell.

- Needlestick injuries as emergency
- Post-exposure prophylaxis (PEP)

A needlestick injury is any injury where the skin has been breached with an infected sharp; this can include grazes as well as puncture injuries (Phillips et al 2011).

Similarly, splashes of blood or blood-stained fluid into the eye are considered to carry the same risk but of a different order. Following a mucocutaneous exposure, via the mucous membrane, the risk of HIV infection is thought to be less than one in one thousand; when intact skin has been exposed to HIV, there is considered to be little to no risk.

### Needlestick injury is an emergency

- Stop what you are doing immediately
- Force the wound to bleed
- Wash under running water
- Report immediately to your immediate manager
- Go directly to Accident & Emergency
- Report to triage nurse, who will award an urgent triage category

### Post-exposure prophylaxis (PEP)

Discuss with A&E clinician whether to commence PEP. PEP standard treatment consists of a combination of three anti-HIV drugs from two different classes. The most recent UK guidelines recommend using Truvada, which is a fixed-dose combination tablet combining emtricitabine and tenofovir, which is prescribed alongside raltegravir.

The course will be of 28 days' duration, and side effects may be experienced, such as tiredness, nausea, sickness and diarrhoea; the side effects are more easily tolerated than previous PEP regimes (National Institute for Health and Care Excellence (NICE)., 2014).

### References

National Institute for Health and Care Excellence (NICE). (2014). *Overview: infection prevention and control.* London: NICE.

Phillips, S., Collins, M., Dougherty, L. (2011). *Venepuncture and cannulation.* Chichester: Wiley Blackwell.

CHAPTER 14
Drug Administration
and Drug Calculation

- Dispensing drugs safely: checklist
- Systeme International
- Making a calculation

The pharmaceutical management of a patient involves two distinct responsibilities and functions, which fall to different professions at different times. These are prescribing the right drug correctly and dispensing the right drug, correctly.

Nurses are now in a position of fulfilling both roles, and historically nurses would encounter drugs as the clinician who dispenses them second to the prescription of a medical colleague. This has now changed in that nurses will often also be the prescriber, since the changes in nurse prescribing came into effect in 2006.

Whatever role the nurse fills, there are many common elements to both functions, namely giving the correct drug to the correct patient for the correct reason.

Whether dispensing or prescribing, it is essential that all the team involved are able to competently calculate and give the right dose (Courtenay & Griffiths 2004).

## Dispensing drugs safely: checklist

Name
Unique identifier (Hospital or NHS number)
DOB
Date
Time
Route
Allergies˙
Drug interactions with other prescribed drugs
Correct dose
Appropriate drug for this patient with this condition

## Systeme International (SI)
### Systeme International (SI) Units

**Mass**

| | |
|---|---|
| 1 kilogram (kg) | 1000 grams |
| 1 gram (g) | 1000 milligrams |
| 1 milligram (mg) | 1000 micrograms |
| 1 microgram ($\mu$g) | 1000 nanograms |

**Volume**

| | |
|---|---|
| 1 litre (L) | 1000 millilitres |
| 1 millilitre (mL) | 1000 microlitres ($\mu$L) |

Abbreviations should not be used in the writing of a prescription, as there is a high possibility of confusion with other prescriptions

## Making a calculation

### First method

This approach allows the nurse to give the correct dose by identifying the strength of the solution per volume; from this point a calculation is undertaken to identify the specific volume needed for the prescribed dose.

**Example 1.** A dose of 100 mg has been prescribed. However, the drug is only available in strengths and volume of 400 mg in 5 mL.

#### Step 1

Calculate the dose per mL:

$$\frac{400\,mg}{5\,mL} = 80\,mg/mL$$

#### Step 2

This preparation therefore has strength of 80 mg per mL.
To achieve a dose of 100 mg, we must do the following calculation:

$$\frac{100\,mg \times 1\,mL}{80\,mg/mL} = 1.25\,mL$$

### Second method

The second method is based on a relationship between proportions.

#### The formula

$$\frac{Dose\ required}{Strength\ available} \times Dose\ volume\ (mL)\ of\ available\ product$$

$$= Volume\ (mL)\ containing\ the\ required\ dose$$

$$\frac{Dose\ required = 100\,mg}{Strength\ available = 400\,mg} \times Dose\ volume\ (mL)\ of\ available\ product = 5$$

$$= 100\,mg\ divided\ by\ 400\,mg = 0.25 \times 5 = 1.25\,mL$$

This formula is most often described as:

$$\frac{What\ you\ want}{What\ you've\ got} \times What\ it's\ in$$

(Davison 2014.)

## References

Courtenay, M., Griffiths, M. (2004). *Independent and supplementary prescribing: an essential guide*. Cambridge: Cambridge University Press.

Davison, N. (2014). *Numeracy and clinical calculations for nurses*. New York: Lantern Publishing.

# CHAPTER 15  Blood Test Interpretation and Values

- Haematology
- Urea and electrolytes
- Liver function tests
- Cardiac enzymes

This chapter details the expected values for a number of the more common blood tests and gives some insight into what low and high values might indicate. This is not intended as a complete and comprehensive interpretation but more a guide in the right direction for the nurse reviewing and ordering these bloods.

## Hematology

| | Range | High | Low |
|---|---|---|---|
| **Hemoglobin (Hb)** | Men: 13–18 g/dL | Polycythaemia Dehydration | Anaemia Blood loss Haemodilution Consider menorrhagia |
| | Women: 11.5–16 g/dL | | |
| **Mean corpuscular volume (MCV)** | 76–96 fL | Alcohol Azathioprine Zidovudine Haemolysis Liver disease Hypothyroid Myelodysplasia Macrocytic anaemia Vitamin $B_{12}$ deficiency Hydroxycarbamide | Microcytic anaemia Poor dietary iron Bleeding |
| **White cell (total)** | WCC 4–11 × $10^9$/L | Possible infection Leukaemia may also increase count | Viral infections Autoimmune diseases Bone marrow infiltration |
| **Neutrophils** | 2–7.5 × $10^9$/L | Viral infections Inflammation Infarction Burns Bleeding Trauma Widespread malignancy Leukaemias | Viral infection Hypersplenism Systemic lupus erythematosus (SLE) Rheumatoid arthritis $B_{12}$ deficiency Folate deficiency Sulfonamides Carbimazole |

| | Range | High | Low |
|---|---|---|---|
| **Lymphocytes** | $1.3–3.5 \times 10^9$/L | Viral infections<br>Toxoplasmosis<br>Whooping cough<br>Chronic lymphocytic<br>leukaemia | SLE<br>Uraemia<br>AIDs<br>Post chemotherapy<br>Post radiotherapy<br>Steroids |
| **Eosinophils** | $0.04–0.44 \times 10^9$/L | Asthma<br>Skin disease<br>(urticarias)<br>Leukaemias<br>Adrenal<br>insufficiency<br>Following infection<br>End organ damage | |
| **Monocytes** | $0.2–0.8 \times 10^9$/L | Acute infections<br>Malignancy<br>Acute myeloid<br>leukaemia<br>Hodgkin disease | |
| **Basophils** | $0.0–10 \times 10^9$/L | Viral infection<br>Malignancy<br>Urticaria<br>Myxoedema<br>Post splenectomy | |
| **Platelets** | $150–400 \times 10^9$/L | Commonly related<br>to infection | Low known as<br>thrombocytopenia<br>Aplastic<br>anaemias<br>Bone marrow<br>infiltration<br>Platelets below 40:<br>there is a<br>greater risk of<br>bleeding |

## Electrolytes

| Electrolyte | Range | High | Low |
|---|---|---|---|
| **Potassium* K+** <br> An erroneously high potassium can be seen in a blood sample that has haemolysed | 3.5–5.0 mmol/L | Oliguric renal failure <br> Excessive K+ therapy <br> Rhabdomyolysis <br> Metabolic acidosis (DM) <br> Addison's disease <br> Large amounts of blood transfusion <br> K+ sparing diuretics <br> ACE inhibitors <br> Suxamethonium | Diuretics <br> D&V <br> Pyloric stenosis <br> GI fistulae <br> Cushing's <br> Alkalosis <br> Renal tubular failure |
| **Sodium** | 135–145 mmol/L | Dehydration, diuretic therapy, renal dysfunction, diarrhoea | Haemodilution, diuretic use, diarrhoea, heart failure, renal disease, liver disease, distribution of anti-diuretic hormone (ADH) |
| **Urea** | 2.5–6.7 mmol/L | Renal insufficiency <br> Haemoconcentration in severe dehydration | Low protein diet <br> Immediately post haemodialysis |
| **Calcium** | 2.12–2.65 mmol/L | Can be found in bone disease | Hypocalcaemia <br> Tetany <br> Neuroexcitability |
| **Albumin** | 35–50 g/L | Dehydration artefact | Nephrotic syndrome <br> Liver disease <br> Malabsorption <br> Malnutrition |
| **Proteins** | 60–80 g/L | As in Albumin | As in Albumin |

*Potassium lower than 2.5 mmol/L needs urgent intervention and is life-threatening. Potassium higher than 6.5 mmol/L needs urgent intervention and is life-threatening.

## Liver function tests (LFTs)

| | Range | High | Low |
|---|---|---|---|
| **Bilirubin** | 3–17 μmol/L | Jaundice likely above 35 | |
| **Alanine aminotransferase** | 3–35 IU/L | Indicates hepatocyte damage | |
| | | Disease of the liver causing jaundice | |
| **Aspartate aminotransferase** | 3–35 IU/L | Indicates hepatocyte damage | |
| | | Disease of the liver causing jaundice | |
| **Alkaline phosphatase** | 30–300 IU/L | May indicate obstructive jaundice but can be present in other conditions such as malignant infiltration | |

(Basten 2019)

## Cardiac enzymes

There are a collection of enzymes and proteins that, when measured, can give useful information on the likelihood of a patient having suffered a myocardial infarction (MI).

The significance of a diagnostic tool to run alongside the ECG is of course important, but this test has a further value in negative values over time and can be a reliable indicator of whether a patient has not suffered an MI.

Troponin T and troponin I increase from 4 to 9 hours after an acute MI, peaking at 12–24 hours, and can remain elevated for up to 14 days. A negative troponin can effectively rule out MI if drawn 12 hours after the onset of symptoms, specifically pain.

## Cardiac enzymes

| | |
|---|---|
| **CK** | Creatine kinase |
| **CK-MB** | CK cardiac isoenzyme |
| **AST** | Aspartate transaminase |
| **LDH** | Lactate dehydrogenase |

CK is found in myocardial muscle and in skeletal muscle, and therefore can be elevated from a non-myocardial source. If in any doubt, measure CK-MB.

CK-MB is a more specific marker for MI and will rise up to 12 hours or so post injury, and will fall away to dissipation by day 3. It is therefore a useful marker for new or subsequent injury (Blann 2013).

#### Enzyme levels and peaks

| | |
|---|---|
| CK can rises to 5 times the normal level | Peaks at day 3 |
| CK-MB can rise to 4 times the normal level | Peaks at day 2 |
| AST can rise to 3 times the normal level | Peaks at day 3 |
| LDH can rise to 3 times the normal level | Peaks at day 3 |

## References

Basten, G. (2019). *Blood results in clinical practice* (2nd edn). Keswick: M&K Publishing.

Blann, A. (2013). *Routine blood results explained*. Keswick: M&K Publishing.

## Further Reading

Forsyth, J.M., Shalan, A., Thompson, A. (2019). *Venous access made easy*. Boca Raton: CRC Press.

## CHAPTER 16

Mental Health and Mental Well-being

- Suicide first aid
- Delirium
- Management of delirium
- Common causes of delirium
- Dementia
- Mini-Mental State Exam
- Nursing care of dementia
- Mental Capacity Act
- Testing capacity
- Best interests
- Children and competency in law

## Suicide

Suicide is the leading cause of death for men under 50 (Sutherland 2018). For such a significant health concern, all nurses should be in a position to deal with patients, clients and people generally that are at risk of suicide.

### Suicide first aid

This section deals with the risk of suicide, and action to take if an individual has demonstrated they may be at risk; if in the initial assessment there is evidence or information about physical harm that is current, such as ingestion of medication as an attempt at overdose, for example, then physical care needs to take priority, whilst maintaining a therapeutic rapport (Sutherland 2018).

| Suicide first aid | |
|---|---|
| Assess the risk | Suicidal ideation |
| | Specific and detailed suicidal narrative |
| | Self-harm |
| | Feeling hopeless |
| | Reckless behaviour |
| | History of previous attempts |
| Listen non-judgementally | Use positive listening skills |
| | Reframe and restate issues |
| | Use positive body posture |
| | Good eye contact |
| Give reassurance and information | Assert a non-blame position |
| | Engender and communicate a sense of dignity and respect |
| | Validate the individual |
| | Recognize the urgent and earnest nature of the problem |
| | Recognize the commonality of the problem |

| Suicide first aid—cont'd | |
|---|---|
| | Empathetically communicate that the individual is not alone |
| | Give information about resources and support available, ensuring that the information is furnished with detailed and specific contacts and instruction |
| Encourage appropriate professional help | Counsellors, doctors, nurses, social workers, etc |
| | Detail the types of help, such as counselling, medication, other professional therapy |
| Encourage self help and other support strategies | Exercise |
| | Relaxation and meditation |
| | Engaging with family and friends – often key family members |
| | Where partners are unaware, support through a meaningful conversation may enable real supportive contact with a key person in the individual's life |

## Delirium

Delirium is a common problem in the hospital environment, with an estimated 5%–15% of all patients in medical and surgical wards suffering with this condition. The condition affects the brain for a short period and is characterized by the seven following signs (Tintinalli et al 2016):

- Impaired consciousness, a sense that the patient is not perceptually engaged fully with the place or the current interaction
- Disoriented to time and place
- Behaviour is altered, can be quiet and withdrawn or irritable, hyperactive and noisy
- Thinking is slow and muddled, often with delusional elements, such as paranoia with accusatory behaviour
- Perception is disturbed and often with illusions and hallucinations
- Mood is labile, anxious, with fear, agitation and depression
- Memory is impaired and can at a later stage be amnesic of this episode

## Management

- Consider differential diagnoses, such as psychogenic-mediated problems
- Identify cause and treat

## Some common causes

- Infection: particularly in the elderly, respiratory or urinary are common sites
- Alcohol withdrawal: should be considered even if the clerking history denies alcohol use
- Drugs such as opiates, sedatives and recreational drug use
- Vascular, such as stroke or transient ischaemic attack (TIA)
- Intracranial infections, such as encephalitis or meningitis

- Trauma with head injury
- Post-ictal epilepsy

## Dementia

There are 850,000 people with dementia in the UK, with that number expected to rise to 1 million by 2025 (alzheimers.org.uk). Dementia is therefore a significant issue for the profession of nursing, as it is for all healthcare professionals. Here described is an assessment tool to identify dementia and key approaches to nursing care of this patient group (Tintinalli et al 2016).

When assessing for dementia, ensure all physical, metabolic and psychological causes of confusion have been ruled out.

---

### Mini-mental state exam

Ask the patient to answer the following questions and complete following tasks:
- What is the year, date, day and month?
- What is the season?
- Where are we (county, town, building, floor)?
- Name three objects, e.g. table, computer, pen. Ask the patient to repeat all three after you have said what they are.
- Say: Please repeat this sentence "No ifs, buts or maybes."
- Show a watch and ask what it is.
- Show a pencil and ask what it is.
- Ask: Please read and do what is said on this piece of paper. The paper should read, "Close your eyes."
- Ask: Write a complete sentence on this paper: The sentence must have a verb and make sense; spelling and grammar are not important.
- Say: Here is a drawing (Fig. 16.1), please copy it. Correct if two figures intersect and all angles are preserved.
- Say: I am going to list three objects different from above, and I would like you to repeat them after me. I also want you to remember them, as I will ask you what they were in a few minutes.
- Say: Now take 7 away from 100 and take 7 away from that number, and keep reducing the number by taking 7 away each time. Every time 7 is correctly taken away, award one 1 point.
- Say: What were the three objects I asked you to remember earlier?

### Interpretation

Maximum score is 30. 25–27 is borderline, and anything below 25 suggests dementia (NICE 2018).

### Nursing care in dementia

#### Key points
- Care should be individualized
- Stimulate and enable
- Include socializing
- Supportive and not challenging

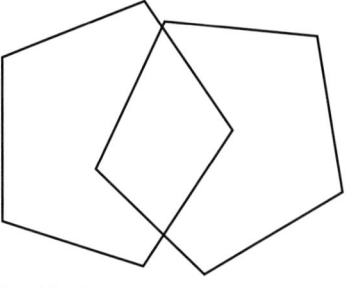

**Fig. 16.1** Mini-mental state examination pentagon copying exercise. (Incalzi, R., Scarlata, S., Pennazza, G., et al. (2014). Chronic obstructive pulmonary disease in the elderly. *European Journal of Internal Medicine*, 25(4), 320–328.)

### Useful interventions
- Memory enhancing
- Use of music
- Reminiscing therapy
- Storytelling therapy
- Object handling
- Singing as therapy
- Environmental modifications to enable a level of independence

These interventions will be alongside medical care and core nursing care.

## Mental Capacity Act 2005

The Mental Capacity Act was enacted in 2005, and it recognizes that the previous legal mechanism could be at times too prescriptive and not allow for a more expansive sense of the individual's ability to make decisions for themselves (Graham & Cowley 2015).

---

### Five principles of the mental capacity act

1. Presumption of capacity
2. Individual supported to make decisions
3. Unwise decisions do not necessarily demonstrate lack of capacity
4. Always do things, or take decisions, for people without capacity in their best interests
5. Before doing something or making a decision for somebody, always consider a less restrictive way

## Testing capacity

In order to decide on whether an individual has the capacity to make a decision, two questions have to be answered:

1. Is there an impairment of, or disturbance in, the functioning of a person's mind or brain?
2. If so, is the impairment or disturbance sufficient that the person lacks capacity to make a particular decision? The impairment or disturbance is sufficient to indicate a lack of capacity if the person concerned cannot do one or more of the following four things:
   - Understand information relevant to the decision
   - Retain that information long enough to be able to make the decision
   - Weigh up pros and cons against own value system
   - Communicate their decision

It is incumbent on the professional assessing capacity that they have a reasonable belief that the individual being assessed does not have capacity.

Following on from an assessment where decisions are being made for an individual, those decisions must be made in the individual's best interests.

## Best interests

A person that makes an unwise decision should not necessarily be treated as being unable to make a decision; it is only when harm to themselves or others is considered likely, or when they are incompetent through some other circumstances such as unconsciousness, that a decision can be made when acting in their best interests.

When a decision is made by a professional, they should be aware and prepared to justify that decision if and when challenged.

## Children and competency in law

In the healthcare environment, if there is a need for a decision regarding consent for care, a child under 16 would have their decision referred to their parents or guardian, as in legal terms they are considered incompetent to make a decision by nature of their age. There is, however, an exception to this, which is Gillick competence. This is where a child can have their capacity to consent assessed and endorsed. This generally runs alongside Fraser guidelines, which are used specifically to decide if a child can consent to sexual health advice or contraception.

## References

Graham, M., Cowley, J. (2015). *A practical guide to the Mental Capacity Act 2005: putting the principles of the Act into practice.* London: Jessica Kingsley Publishers.

National Institute for Health and Care Excellence (NICE). (2018). *Dementia: assessment, management and support for people living with dementia and their carers* [NG97]. London: NICE.

Sutherland, R. (2018). *Tackling the root cause of suicide.* NHS England. Available at: https://www.england.nhs.uk/blog/tackling-the-root-causes-of-suicide/

Tintinalli, J.E., Stapczynski, S., Ma, O.J., et al. (2016). *Tintinalli's Emergency Medicine: A Comprehensive Study Guide* (8th edn). New York: McGraw-Hill.

# CHAPTER 17 Paediatric Considerations

- Paediatric nursing
- Vital signs in children
- NICE guidelines for temperature recording National Institute for Health and Care Excellence (NICE)., 2019
- Resuscitation: Basic Paediatric Life Support algorithm
- Paediatric resuscitation
- Paediatric resuscitation and size
- Resuscitation: Advanced Paediatric Life Support algorithm

## Paediatric nursing

Nursing care of children differs from all other types of nursing because of the different context and importance of family, play, development, size and physiological reserve. Here follows some guidance on the nursing care and management of the child, with a focus on the challenges and difference presented by the physiology and anatomy of the child (Ajithkumar 2018).

## Vital signs and normal values in children

### Normal heart rate by age (beats/minute)

| Age | Awake range | Sleeping range |
|---|---|---|
| Neonate (<28 days) | 100–205 | 90–160 |
| Infant (1 month–1 year) | 100–190 | 90–160 |
| Toddler (1–2 years) | 98–140 | 80–120 |
| Preschool (3–5 years) | 80–120 | 65–100 |
| School age (6–11 years) | 75–118 | 58–90 |
| Adolescent (12–15 years) | 60–100 | 50–90 |

### Normal respiratory rate by age (breaths/minute)

| Age | Awake range |
|---|---|
| Infant (<1 year) | 30–53 |
| Toddler (1–2 years) | 22–37 |
| Preschool (3–5 years) | 20–28 |
| School age (6–11 years) | 18–25 |
| Adolescent (12–15 years) | 12–20 |

### Normal blood pressure by age (measured in mmHg)

| Age | Systolic pressure | Diastolic |
|---|---|---|
| Neonate (<28 days) | 67–84 | 35–53 |
| Infant (1 month–1 year) | 72–104 | 37–56 |
| Toddler (1–2 years) | 86–106 | 42–63 |
| Preschool (3–5 years) | 89–112 | 46–72 |

| Age | Systolic pressure | Diastolic |
|---|---|---|
| School age (6–9 years) | 97–115 | 57–76 |
| Adolescent (10–11 years) | 102–120 | 61–80 |
| Adolescent (12–15 years) | 110–131 | 64–83 |

**Normal temperature by method**

| Method | Temperature (°C) |
|---|---|
| Rectal | 36.6–38.0 |
| Ear | 35.8–38.0 |
| Oral | 35.5–37.5 |
| Axillary | 36.5–37.5 |

### The NICE guideline (NG143) for temperature recording in children

- 0–4 weeks: electronic thermometer at axilla
- 4 weeks to 5 years: electronic thermometer at axilla, chemical dot at axilla or infra-red tympanic thermometer
- Avoid oral or rectal route in children
- Avoid forehead dot thermometers, as unreliable National Institute for Health and Care Excellence (NICE)., 2019

### Resuscitation guidelines

### Basic paediatric life support 2021 (Fig. 17.1)

### Paediatric resuscitation

The resuscitation of children is different from adult resuscitation because the respiratory system is the priority, as children invariably have a respiratory-mediated event, whereas adults generally have a cardiac-mediated event.

The implication for resuscitation is that the child will invariably have depleted the oxygen in the blood stream, as respiration prior to arrest would have been insufficient; therefore, it is necessary to begin resuscitation with 5 rescue breaths with a cycle of 15:2, giving greater opportunity for oxygenation (Resuscitation Council UK RCUK., 2021).

#### *Considerations with paediatric resuscitation*

Begin with 5 rescue breaths.

In chest compressions, the chest should be compressed by a third: 4 cm in an infant, 5 cm in an older child.

Airway management is different in the child as their anatomy is different. For the infant, the head should be in a neutral position to avoid overextension and the potential of collapsing the airway.

The rescue breath is applied by creating a seal over both the nose and the mouth, which is achieved by the use of an oxygen mask covering both.

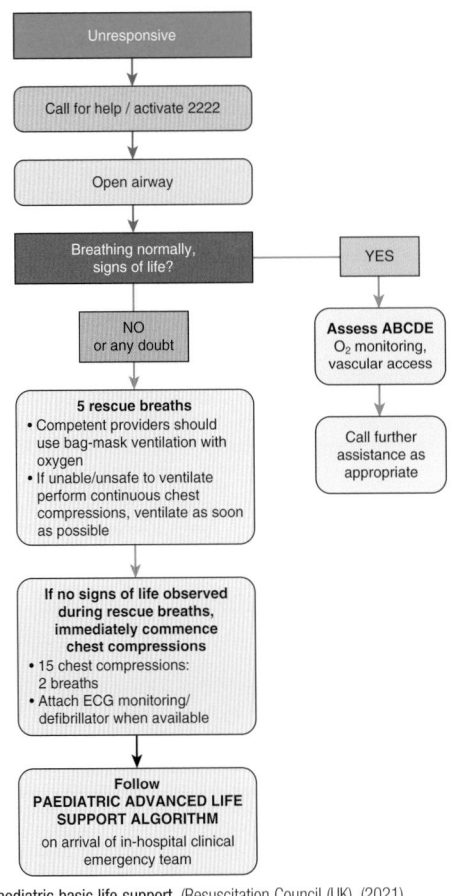

**Paediatric basic life support**

Unresponsive

Call for help / activate 2222

Open airway

Breathing normally, signs of life?

YES

NO or any doubt

**Assess ABCDE**
O₂ monitoring, vascular access

Call further assistance as appropriate

**5 rescue breaths**
- Competent providers should use bag-mask ventilation with oxygen
- If unable/unsafe to ventilate perform continuous chest compressions, ventilate as soon as possible

**If no signs of life observed during rescue breaths, immediately commence chest compressions**
- 15 chest compressions: 2 breaths
- Attach ECG monitoring/ defibrillator when available

**Follow PAEDIATRIC ADVANCED LIFE SUPPORT ALGORITHM**
on arrival of in-hospital clinical emergency team

**Fig. 17.1** Paediatric basic life support. (Resuscitation Council (UK). (2021). Paediatric Basic Life Support. Available at: https://www.resus.org.uk/library/2021-resuscitation-guidelines/paediatric-bas ic-life-support-guidelines.)

The child's airway is opened with a manoeuvre where the head is positioned in a modified and reduced head tilt, chin lift, where they are placed into a position described as *sniffing the morning air*.

## Paediatric resuscitation and considerations of size

When resuscitating a child (Paediatric Advanced Life Support; Fig. 17.2), there is a specific need to quantify weight so that the following are correctly calculated (RCUK 2021):

- Energy for defibrillation
- Dosage of drugs
- Volumes of fluid

This information can be calculated by using instructions which are described in the WETFLAG mnemonic (Resuscitation Council UK RCUK., 2021):

**W**eight = (age + 4) × 2. Estimated weight of child

**E**nergy = 4 × weight (J) – the energy required for defibrillation

**T**ube = age/4 + 4 (approximate size of uncuffed endotracheal tube to use for intubation)

**F**luids = 20 mL/kg of N/saline bolus

**A**drenaline = 10 mcg/kg = 0.1 mL/kg of adrenaline 1:10,000

**G**lucose = 2 mL/kg of 10% glucose

## References

Ajithkumar, D. (2018). *Introduction to paediatric nursing*. Kerala: Government College of Nursing.

National Institute for Health and Care Excellence (NICE). (2019). *Fever in under 5s: Assessment and initial management* [NG143]. London: NICE. Available at: https://www.nice.org.uk/guidance/ng143/resources/fever-in-under-5s-assessment-and-initial-management-pdf-66141778137541

Resuscitation Council (UK) (RCUK). (2021). *Resuscitation guidelines 2021: paediatric advanced life support*. London: RCUK.

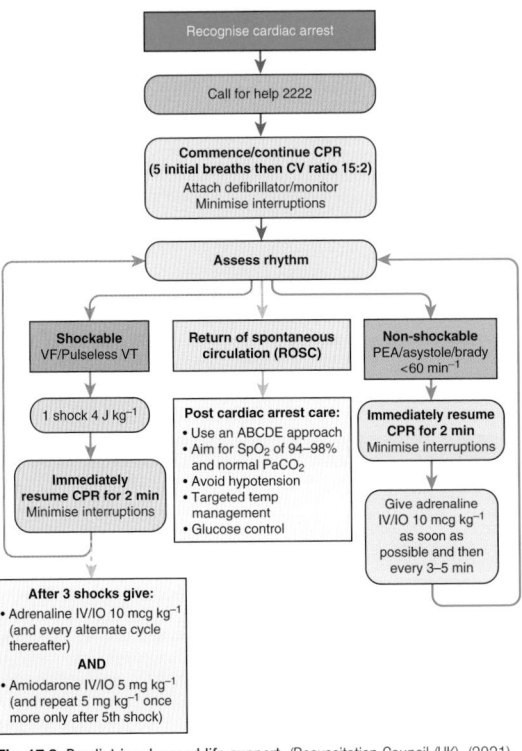

**Fig. 17.2** Paediatric advanced life support. (Resuscitation Council (UK). (2021). Paediatric Advanced Life Support. Available at: https://www.resus.org.uk/library/2015-resuscitation-guidelines/paediatric-advanced-life-support)

| During CPR | Identify and treat reversible causes |
|---|---|

**During CPR**

- **Ensure high quality chest compressions are delivered:**
  – Correct rate, depth and full recoil
- Provide BMV with 100% oxygen (2 person approach)
- Provide continuous chest compressions when a tracheal tube is in place.
- Competent providers can consider an advanced airway and capnography, and ventilate at a rate (breaths minute$^{-1}$) of:

**Identify and treat reversible causes**

- Hypoxia
- Hypovolaemia
- Hyperkalaemia, hypercalcaemia, hypermagnesemia, hypoglycaemia
- Hypo-/hyperthermia
- Thrombosis – coronary or pulmonary
- Tension pneumothorax
- Tamponade – cardiac
- Toxic agents

Adjust algorithm in specific settings (e.g. special circumstances)

| Infants: 25 | 1–8 years: 20 | 8–12 years: 15 | > 12 years: 10–12 |
|---|---|---|---|

- Vascular access IV/IO
- Once started, give Adrenaline every 3–5 min
- Maximum single dose Adrenaline 1 mg
- Maximum single dose Amiodarone 300 mg

**Fig. 17.2, cont'd**

# CHAPTER 18 Safeguarding

- Five types of abuse
- Prevention management

Safeguarding is a fundamental concern of all healthcare professionals in that preventing harm is a priority above resolving problems of health. Safeguarding is the prevention of harm, particularly in the extreme risk of abuse.

Abuse occurs when one person sets out to hurt, harm, damage or exploit another (Cooper & White 2017).

## Five types of abuse

- Physical
- Emotional
- Sexual
- Financial
- Neglect

## Signs of physical abuse

- Cuts, bruises, fractures
- Poor skin condition
- Soiled bedding
- Signs of restraint
- Inappropriate use of medication

## Emotional abuse: warning signs and behaviours

- Belittling, threatening or controlling behavior by the caregiver
- In the elderly, the patient may demonstrate behavior that mimics dementia, such as rocking, sucking or mumbling to themselves

## Signs of sexual abuse

- Bruising around breasts or genitals
- Unexplained vaginal or anal bleeding
- Underclothing stained, bloody or torn

## Signs of financial abuse

- Unusual financial behaviour, large amounts withdrawn from bank account
- Sudden change in financial circumstances of the patient
- Cash or items missing from the patient's home
- Sudden unexpected change in the patient's will
- Unnecessary goods or services being ordered
- Behaviour that is at odds with the patient's circumstances, such as cash withdrawals from ATM machine when the patient is immobile

## Signs of neglect

- Problems of weight loss, malnutrition and dehydration

- Physical problems, such bed sores, that are untreated and not highlighted to healthcare staff
- Unsanitary home conditions with dirty or soiled bedclothes
- Dressed inappropriately for the season
- Infrastructural shortfalls with electricity or heating not working properly
- Being deserted in public places

(See Lindon 2012.)

## Prevention and management

- Support of the caregiver, particularly in the home environment where social isolation is highly possibility
- Education of healthcare staff to identify abuse; Protection of Vulnerable Adult (POVA) training is mandatory in many health and social care environments
- Screening of healthcare staff with checks such as the Disclosure and Barring Service (DBS) check
- Referral, debarring and criminal sanction of individuals who have been responsible for abuse

## References

Cooper, A., White, E. (2017). *Safeguarding adults under the care act 2014: Understanding good practice.* London: Jessica Kingsley Publishers.

Lindon, J. (2012). *Safeguarding and child protection: 0–8 years* (4th edn). London: Hodder Education.

# CHAPTER 19 Pressure Area Care

- Assessment: who's at risk?
- Assessment: the skin
- Waterlow scoring system
- Actions and interventions

Pressure area care is a fundamental concern of the nurse, as many, possibly all, patients have some level of vulnerability to pressure area injury, even the seemingly low-risk, mobile patient who enjoys good nutrition.

## Assessment: who's at risk?

- Limited mobility
- Previous pressure ulcer
- Malnutrition and dehydration
- The inability to reposition themselves
- Cognitive impairment
- Remember: risk changes: for example, a fit, mobile patient in a state of good nutrition when anaesthetized and immobile in an operating theatre will be significantly at risk

## Assessment: the skin

- Poor skin integrity at point of potential pressure
- Colour changes or discolouration
- Exposure to body fluids, through incontinence or wound leakage

## Waterlow scoring system

Fig. 19.1 represents a pressure ulcer risk assessment tool. It is based on the Waterlow assessment, which is the most used in the UK healthcare environment.

The process allows an evaluation of patients who present a potential for developing pressure sores, where the aggregate score will direct the nurse to planning the most appropriate interventions. The original tool, the Waterlow Score, was devised by Judy Waterlow in 1985, and updated in 2015 (Waterlow 2015).

### Score interpretation

- 9 or less: Patient presents little to no risk
- 10–14: Patient is at risk
- 15–19: Patient is at high risk
- 20 and above: Patient is at very high risk

### Actions and intervention

- Encourage or enable regular repositions of patient
- Ensure good nutrition and hydration, giving supplements if necessary
- Avoid subcutaneous fluids
- Use a high-quality pressure distribution mattress
- Air mattress
- Barrier creams, particularly in instances of soiling and incontinence
- Mobilizing in all healthcare is the key to improving outcome

(NICE 2020)

The Waterlow score

# WATERLOW PRESSURE ULCER PREVENTION/TREATMENT POLICY
RING SCORES IN TABLE, ADD TOTAL. MORE THAN 1 SCORE/CATEGORY CAN BE USED

| BUILD/WEIGHT FOR HEIGHT | ◆ | SKIN TYPE VISUAL RISK AREAS | ◆ | SEX AGE | ◆ | MALNUTRITION SCREENING TOOL (MST) (Nutrition Vol. 15, No. 6 1999 – Australia) | | |
|---|---|---|---|---|---|---|---|---|
| AVERAGE BMI = 20-24.9 | 0 | HEALTHY | 0 | MALE | 1 | A – HAS PATIENT LOST WEIGHT RECENTLY | | B – WEIGHT LOSS SCORE |
| ABOVE AVERAGE BMI = 25-29.9 | 1 | TISSUE PAPER | 1 | FEMALE | 2 | YES – GO TO B | | 0.5–5 kg = 1 |
| OBESE BMI > 30 | 2 | DRY | 1 | 14–49 | 1 | NO – GO TO C | | 5–10 kg = 2 |
| BELOW AVERAGE BMI < 20 | 3 | OEDEMATOUS | 1 | 50–64 | 2 | UNSURE – GO TO C AND SCORE 2 | | 10–15 kg = 3 |
| BMI = Wt(kg)/Ht(m)² | | CLAMMY, PYREXIA | 1 | 65–74 | 2 | | | >15 kg = 4 |
| | | DISCOLOURED GRADE 1 | 2 | 75–80 | 3 | | | unsure = 2 |
| | | BROKEN/SPOTS GRADE 2-4 | 3 | 81+ | 5 | C – PATIENT EATING POORLY OR LACK OF APPETITE 'NO' = 0; 'YES' SCORE = 1 | | NUTRITION SCORE If > 2 refer for nutrition assessment / intervention |

| CONTINENCE | ◆ | MOBILITY | ◆ | SPECIAL RISKS | | |
|---|---|---|---|---|---|---|
| COMPLETE/ CATHETERISED | 0 | FULLY | 0 | TISSUE MALNUTRITION | ◆ | NEUROLOGICAL DEFICIT | ◆ |
| URINE INCONT. | 1 | RESTLESS/FIDGETY | 1 | TERMINAL CACHEXIA | 8 | DIABETES, MS, CVA | 4–6 |
| FAECAL INCONT. | 2 | APATHETIC | 2 | MULTIPLE ORGAN FAILURE | 8 | MOTOR/SENSORY | 4–6 |
| URINARY + FAECAL INCONTINENCE | 3 | RESTRICTED | 3 | SINGLE ORGAN FAILURE (RESP, RENAL, CARDIAC) | 5 | PARAPLEGIA (MAX OF 6) | 4–6 |
| | | BEDBOUND e.g. TRACTION | 4 | PERIPHERAL VASCULAR DISEASE | 5 | MAJOR SURGERY or TRAUMA | |
| | | CHAIRBOUND e.g. WHEELCHAIR | 5 | ANAEMIA (HB < 8) | 2 | ORTHOPAEDIC/SPINAL | 5 |
| | | | | SMOKING | 1 | ON TABLE > 2 HR# | 5 |
| | | | | | | ON TABLE > 6 HR# | 8 |

MEDICATION – CYTOTOXICS, LONG TERM/HIGH DOSE STEROIDS, ANTI-INFLAMMATORY MAX OF 4

| SCORE |
|---|
| 10+ AT RISK |
| 15+ HIGH RISK |
| 20+ VERY HIGH RISK |

#Scores can be discounted after 48 hours provided patient is recovering normally

Fig. 19.1 The waterlow score.

## References

National Institute for Health and Care Excellence (NICE). (2020). *Pressure ulcers, prevention and management* [CG179]. London: NICE. Available at: https://www.nice.org.uk/guidance/cg179

Waterlow, J. (2015). *The Waterlow pressure ulcer prevention manual.* Available at: http://www.judy-waterlow.co.uk.

## Further Reading

Perry, A.G., Potter, P.A., Ostendorf, W.R. (2019). *Clinical nursing skills & techniques* (9th edn). St Louis: Elsevier.

Raison, N., Alwan, W., Abbot, A., Lawton, K. (2012). Improving the management of pressure ulcer care in fracture neck of femur patients RSS. *International Journal of Surgery,* 10(8), S61–S62.

- Good technique
- Practice to be avoided
- Communication
- Manual handling and the law
- MHOR key priorities
- Reduction of risk: TILE
- Manual handling issues for management

Manual handling is a core skill for all healthcare workers, but particularly the nurse who is exposed most frequently to this potentially dangerous activity. It should be noted that in excess of 30% of all workplace injuries reported to the Health and Safety Executive are related to moving and handling.

This chapter describes some useful resources and techniques to improve safety for the individual nurse as well as for the whole healthcare team.

## Good technique

- Position yourself with a good stable base before attempting a moving and handling manoeuvre
- Legs apart
- Knees slightly bent
- Back straight
- Close to the patient you are about to move

## To be avoided

- Never attempt a patient-handling manoeuvre when off balance
- Do not extend or rotate spine
- The patient, or any load, when being moved should be held close to the body
- Never carry out a manual handling manoeuvre in front of the knees or to one side of them
- The vertical dead lift should be avoided

## Communication

- Each manoeuvre should have a team leader
- Ensure the patient fully understands what is about to happen so as to avoid a sudden movement from a surprised patient mid-procedure
- Ensure all members of staff understand what is planned
- Achieve a consensus on the command that is to be used and use a command that carries an implicit instruction with it, such as: 'Ready, steady, slide' or 'Ready, steady, roll'

## Manual handling and the law

Manual handling is a function subject to the law, as it is a workplace activity than can expose staff to harm and risk of injury.

## Legislation that covers moving and handling

- The Health and Safety at Work Act (1974)
- The Management of Health and Safety at Work Act (1992)
- Manual Handling Operations Regulations (MHOR) (1992)
- The Management of Health and Safety at Work Regulations (1999)

## MHOR key principles

- Avoidance
- Assessment
- Reduction of risk
- Review of risk

### Avoidance

- Ensure equipment, such as a patient hoist, is in place to avoid lifting
- Ensure local culture supports use of correct technique and approach to moving and handling
- Redesign processes that insist on unnecessary moving and handling, for example preoperative, pre-anaesthetic patients being lifted unnecessarily in operative department
- Ensure rotation of staff in areas of high exposure to moving and handling

### Assessment

- Use a structure assessment tool such TILE (discussed later in this chapter)
- Assess each patient, including a record in the nursing record where appropriate
- In environments where the patient visit is transitory, it may be more appropriate to assess a process and construct planning according

### Reduction of risk

- Use the assessment plan when planning moving and handling
- Maintain and use equipment
- Encourage the correct culture and approach to risk relevant to this activity
- Regularly review processes as environment and people change

## Tile

TILE is an acronym that guides the assessment process and ensures a consistent and comprehensive approach.

T = Task
I = Individual capacity
L = Load
E = Environment

## Task: note the following in your assessment

- Holding away from trunk
- Stooping
- Reaching upwards
- Lifting and lowering
- Carrying for long distances
- Strenuous pushing or pulling
- Unpredictability of load
- Repetitive handling: are there recovery periods?

- A work rate imposed by a process
- Insufficient rest or recovery periods

### Individual capacity: note the following in your assessment
- Hazardous to those with a health problem
- Hazardous to pregnant women
- Calls for special information or training
- Is movement or posture hindered by clothing or personal protective equipment?

### Load: note the following in your assessment
- Heavy
- Bulky or unwieldy
- Difficult to grasp
- Unstable or unpredictable
- Intrinsically harmful – sharp or hot

### Environment: note the following in your assessment
- Constraints on posture
- Poor floor surface
- Variations in levels
- Hot, cold or humid conditions
- Strong air movement
- Poor lighting conditions

### Manual handling – issues of management
- Training – ensure a regular process of annual training updates
- Assessment – undertake regular assessment and ensure good documentary template available to staff
- Equipment and beds – ensure beds and all equipment regularly serviced and fit for purpose
- Staffing – adequate staff numbers that increase with workload
- Adequate rest breaks – enable a culture where breaks are routine
- Accident reporting – reporting and auditing accidents enables identification and resolution of problems (Nelson 2009)

### Vulnerable staff

When responsible for a group of staff, vulnerability of certain groups must be considered and specifically managed:
- Ageing
- History of direct trauma
- Congenital defects
- Pregnancy
- Diabetes and other systemic disorders
- Upper limb disorders

## References

Nelson, A.L., Motacki, K., Menzel, N. (2009). *The Illustrated guide to safe patient handling and movement*. New York: Springer.

## Further Reading

Dougherty, L., Lister, S. (2011). *The Royal Marsden manual of clinical nursing procedures* (8th edn). Oxford: Oxford University Press.

Price, J., Bowker, L., Shah, K.S., Smith, S. (2006). *Oxford handbook of geriatric medicine* (3rd edn). Oxford: Oxford University Press.

Roffey, D., Wai, E.K., Bishop, P., et al. (2010). Causal assessment of workplace manual handling or assisting patients and low back pain. *The Spine Journal*, 10(7), 639–651.

- Bristol stool chart
- Management of an outbreak of diarrhoea and vomiting
- Constipation
- Urinary incontinence and urinary catheter
- Urinary catheter in acute setting
- Urinary incontinence management
- Devices and surgery

Core to the role of the nurse is the management and maintenance of the patient's processes of elimination – defecation and micturition. Given the intimate and personal nature of these functions, it is of course incumbent on the nurse to ensure that the patient's dignity and privacy are maintained at all times.

When discussing bowel motions it is very important to share information that is understood by all colleagues. This comes into particularly sharp focus when dealing with an outbreak of diarrhoea infection, when the description of the stool is key to the management; this is the rationale for the widely used Bristol stool chart (Fig. 21.1) (Kennedy et al 2018).

### Managing an outbreak of diarrhea and vomiting

Diarrhoea is generally described as type 6–7 on the Bristol stool chart.
- Identify source
- Isolate and barrier nurse
- Treat infected patient/s
- Terminally clean
- Close ward until infection free

### Constipation

#### Possible causes

- Drug history, particularly opiates
- Neurological concurrency
- Thyroid insufficiency
- Poor diet with high amounts of processed food and poor vegetable and fibre intake
- Poor fluid intake
- Inflammatory bowel disorder
- Psychological and behavioural problems
- Socially mediated problems, such as lack of privacy or reduced mobility

#### Management options

- Lifestyle counselling, for dietary problems
- Actuate social manoeuvres if social problems are the cause
- Modify or change analgesia; may need input of pain specialist

**Bristol Stool Chart**

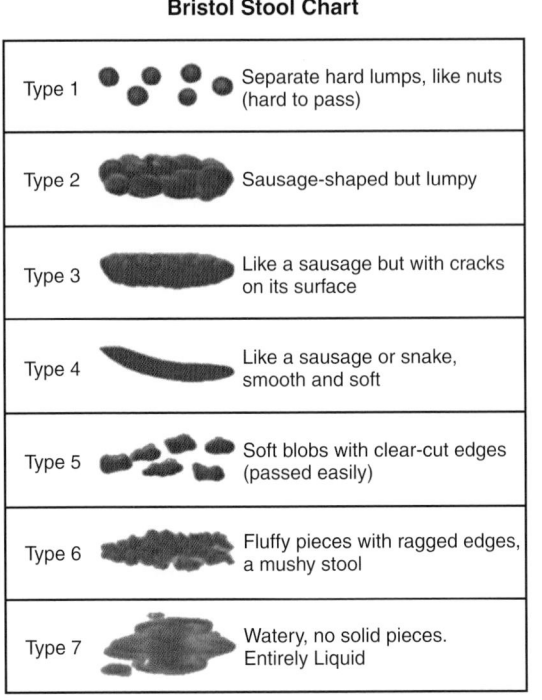

| | | |
|---|---|---|
| Type 1 | | Separate hard lumps, like nuts (hard to pass) |
| Type 2 | | Sausage-shaped but lumpy |
| Type 3 | | Like a sausage but with cracks on its surface |
| Type 4 | | Like a sausage or snake, smooth and soft |
| Type 5 | | Soft blobs with clear-cut edges (passed easily) |
| Type 6 | | Fluffy pieces with ragged edges, a mushy stool |
| Type 7 | | Watery, no solid pieces. Entirely Liquid |

**Fig. 21.1** The Bristol stool chart. (Elder, J. (2020). Enuresis and voiding dysfunction. In: Kliegman, R., St. Geme, J., Blum, N., et al (eds). *Textbook of Pediatrics* (21st edn) (pp. 2816–2821). Philadelphia: Elsevier.)

- Medical options:
  - Bulk-forming agents
  - Emollient stool softeners
  - Prokinetics
  - Osmotic laxatives
  - Enema
  - Suppositories

## The urinary catheter and urinary incontinence

Urinary catheters are used for a number of reasons (Siroky et al 2004). In the acute environment they are primarily used to:

- Enable an accurate fluid balance measurement
- Manage incontinence where the patient is immobile; this is usually achieved as a secondary benefit following the primary want of fluid management observation, as an indwelling urinary catheter is a portal by which infection can enter the sterile environment of the bladder
- Medication such as chemotherapy can be given via a catheter in order to treat cancers topically in that area

### Urinary catheter nursing care

- Regular catheter care should be carried out
- Good volumes of fluid need to be encouraged to maintain good outflow of urine preventing stasis and opportunity for bacteria to collect
- Ensure the collection bag is always below the level of the bladder to avoid backflow and risk of infection that entails
- Regularly change catheter bag and tubing
- An appropriate catheter should be selected for the purpose needed; that is, a long-term silicone catheter should be selected for long-term use

### Urinary incontinence management

- In collaboration with the patient, take a urinary voiding diary
- Treat concurrent problems such as constipation; also rule out and manage urinary tract infection
- Bladder training and pelvic floor exercises
- Double voiding, where a patient is encouraged to void their bladder again shortly after the first, can help to reduce residual urine
- Dietary and fluid management, for example reducing caffeine and alcohol intake
- Anticholinergics for overactive bladder
- Beta-3 agonist such as mirabegron, which also helps overactive bladder
- Alpha blockers, particularly for men with problems related to benign prostatic hypertrophy
- Topical oestrogen in women, which helps rejuvenate local tissue and tone

### Devices and surgery

- Urethral insert, particularly useful prior to an activity such as sport, which may correlate with a worsening of symptoms
- Pessary ring, where incontinence is found with prolapse
- Bulking agents injected around the urethra
- Bladder sling, used to lift and support the urethra
- Botox locally to the bladder muscle to reduce overactivity
- Artificial sphincter, which is a passive device placed that increases resistance allowing the bladder to fill before voiding

## References

Kennedy, M., Martin, P., Duffy, L., Groenke, E. (2018). *Advanced practice nursing in the care of older adults*. Philadelphia: F.A. Davies.

Siroky, M.B., Oates, R.D., Babayan, R.K. (2004). *Handbook of urology: diagnosis and therapy*. Philadelphia: Lippincott.

## Further Reading

Sinclair, A.J., Morley, J.E., Vellas, B., et al. (2012). *Pathy's principles and practice of geriatric medicine*. Hoboken: Wiley-Blackwell.

- Standard precautions
- The spread of infection
- Hospital-acquired infection
- Bacteria and spread of infection
- Hand washing
- MRSA

Infection control is a key concern for all professionals involved with patient care. The following are the key issues and key interventions for the control of infection.

## Standard precautions

Standard precautions are a method in clinical practice that recognizes that all body products from all patients constitute a risk, and therefore stipulates the use of a barrier between the nurse and all body products. This protocol is followed with all patients, which provides a consistent approach, thereby maintaining patient confidentiality, as the nurse's behaviour does not change even in the presence of a known infection (Weston et al 2016).

## The spread of infection

The spread of infection is often referred to as the chain of infection due to the interlinked sequence of events.

---

### Chain of infection

- A causal agent – the organism responsible
- A reservoir – hospital equipment
- A portal of entry – where the skin integrity is compromised, for example at the site of an infusion
- A mode of transmission – from the hand of the attendant nurse
- A portal of exit – the point of contact

Breaking this chain of events at any point will result in an effective reduction in the incidence of infection.

## Hospital-acquired infection

In a recent survey, 5.5% of the hospital population were found to be suffering from a hospital-acquired infection (Mackley et al 2018); that is a significant number of patients who have incurred great risk to health whilst being treated for another condition. This is a compelling mandate for a robust policy of infection control.

Hospital patients are prone to acquire infection due to:
- Invasive procedures
- Patient vulnerability due to underlying conditions
- Prolonged hospital stays, which effectively prolong exposure to other organisms resident in that environment

## Bacteria and the spread of infection

There are always micro-organisms resident on the skin of the hands, which can be classified into two broadly defined types that behave differently and have different implications for our approach to infection control. These two groups are resident and transient.

### Types of micro-organism

| Resident | Transient |
| --- | --- |
| Deep seated | Superficial |
| Difficult to remove | Transfer with ease |
| Part of body's natural defence system | An important source of cross infection |
| Associated with infection following surgery | Easily removed with good hand washing |

Good hand washing removes both resident and superficial bacteria, but particular effort is needed to remove the deep-seated bacteria, for example in preparation for surgery.

### Hand washing

Washing your hands properly should take around 40-60 seconds. Use the steps shown in Fig. 22.1 from the World Health Organization.

Gloves should be used in any intervention where you might be exposed to body fluids. However, hand washing should still be observed meticulously, as moisture caused by wearing gloves encourages bacterial growth on the skin of the hand.

When undertaking clinical procedures, ensure that appropriate facilities are close at hand for appropriate disposal of clinical waste so that this potential source of infection is not moved around unnecessarily.

### Methicillin-resistant *staphylococcus aureus* (MRSA)

It has been estimated that of the 33% of the population that are colonized with *Staphylococcus aureus,* 1% of that number are MRSA positive (Weston et al 2016); in the UK, that is more than 200,000 people. This significant number represents significant risk and a considerable responsibility to nurses and healthcare workers to protect our patient population from an infection that is increasingly difficult to treat.

### Proactive management of MRSA

- Consider every source contaminated
- Isolate all new admissions to care environments until proven negative for MRSA carriage
- Pre-admission screening
- If at all possible, manage patients away from healthcare environment if known positive
- Have robust processes of screening
  - Three consecutive negative screens
  - Each swab taken on different days
  - Swabs from more than one site on each screening

**Wash hands only when visibly soiled! Otherwise use handrub!**

 Duration of the entire procedure: 40–60 sec.

| | | |
|---|---|---|
|  1 |  2 |  3 |
| Wet hands with water using elbow-operated or non-touch taps (if available) | Apply enough soap to cover all hand surfaces | Rub hands palm to palm |

| | | |
|---|---|---|
|  7 |  8 |  9 |
| Rotational rubbing of left thumb clasped in right palm and vice versa | Rotational rubbing, backwards and forwards with clasped fingers of right hand in left palm and vice versa | Rinse hands with water |

| | | |
|---|---|---|
|  4 |  5 |  6 |
| Right palm over left dorsum with interlaced fingers and vice versa | Palm to palm with fingers interlaced | Backs of fingers to opposing palms with fingers interlaced |

| | | |
|---|---|---|
|  10 |  11 |  12 |
| Dry thoroughly with a single-use towel | If hand-operated taps have been used, use towel to turn off tap | ...and your hands are clean |

**Fig. 22.1** World Health Organization (WHO) guidelines on hand hygiene in healthcare (adapted). (Sandoe, J., Dockrell, D. (2018). Principles of infectious disease. In: *Davidson's Principles and Practice of Medicine* (23rd edn) (pp. 99–129). Edinburgh: Elsevier.)

**When MRSA has been identified in an environment**

- Identify source
- Isolate and barrier nurse
- Treat infected patient/s
- Terminally clean
- Close ward until infection free

## References

Mackley, A., Baker, C., Bate, A. (2018). *Raising standards of infection prevention and control in the NHS.* London: House of Commons Liberary.

Weston, D., Burgess, A., Roberts, S. (2016). *Infection prevention and control at a glance.* Chichester: Wiley Blackwell.

## Further Reading

Dougherty, L., Lister, S. (1991). *The Royal Marsden manual of clinical nursing procedures* (9th edn). Chichester: Wiley Blackwell.

Horton, & Parker, R. (2002). *Informed infection control practice.* Edinburgh: Churchill Livingstone.

National Institute for Health and Care Excellence (NICE). (2014). *Infection prevention and control* [QS61]. London: NICE.

## CHAPTER 23

**Care and Cultural Needs at the Time of the Patient's Death**

- Christian faith
- Hinduism
- Judaism
- Islam
- Buddhism
- Sikhism

When practising in multicultural and multi-faith communities, it is important to recognize faith as a core concern to the patient and their family, and that at the time of death certain considerations and religious practice might need to be observed.

Good end-of-life care planning will direct engagement with the patient and the family ahead of an expected death so that any necessary arrangements can be planned ahead of time. The following are some major religions with descriptions of religious practices at time of death (Saccomano & Abbatiello 2014).

---

**Religious practices at time of death**

| | |
|---|---|
| **Christianity** | Practices can vary in different denominations of Christianity. |
| | Roman Catholics often request sacrament of penance, anointing of the sick, and holy communion at the end of life. |
| | Protestants receive sacraments of holy communion or sometimes baptism. |
| | There is no specific prescribed ritual for the preparation of the body. In most cases, post-mortem and organ donation are permissible. |
| **Hinduism** | The head of the person nearing death should face east with a light source near the head. Chanting of the Mantra happens as death approaches, and if the dying person cannot manage, a relative can undertake this for them, chanting into their right ear. |
| | Passages from the *Bhagavad Gita* are recited. |
| | Members of the family prefer to wash the body after death and will chant, pray and use incense. |
| | Hindus prefer to avoid post-mortem and organ donation unless compelled by law. |
| **Judaism** | Traditionally in orthodox Judaism, as the death approaches, there will be reading from the Torah, and often deathbed confessional and blessing. |
| | A family member stays with the body until burial. The eyes of the deceased are closed by a family member. The body is wrapped in white linen. |
| | Burial takes place within 24 hours. |
| | Organ donation and post-mortem may be prohibited in orthodoxy unless compelled by law. |

| Religious practices at time of death—cont'd | |
|---|---|
| **Islam** | As death approaches, a Muslim reader will recite verses from the Qur'an. |
| | The body is prepared by the family, and non-Muslims should not touch the body. |
| | Organ donation and post-mortem are prohibited unless compelled by law |
| **Buddhism** | When death has occurred, cover the body with a cotton sheet, leaving mouth and eyes open. |
| | Strict silence should be maintained after death. |
| | Post-mortem and organ donation are permitted. |
| **Sikhism** | As the patient is dying, the family may request hymns are sung from the holy book; a Sikh priest may also be requested. |
| | The Sikhs believe the material body has only significance for carriage of the immortal soul and therefore have no real objections to organ donation and post-mortem. |
| | Cremation is preferred but not mandatory. |
| | The deceased body can be touched by non-Sikhs; however, males only are requested to touch male deceased, and females correspondingly. |

(De Souza and Pettifer 2016)

## Some general considerations

- One should not assume cultural and religious practices, as individuals may differ from what is expected or may not adhere so specifically.
- The deceased are subject to the law, and the coroner has legal priority when it comes to issues such as post-mortem and when a body may be released for burial.

## References

De Souza, J., Pettifer, A. (2016). *End of life nursing care: a guide for best practice.* London: Sage.
Saccomano, S., Abbatiello, G. (2014). Cultural considerations at the end of life. *The Nurse Practitioner,* 39(2), 24–31.

## Further Reading

Murray Parkes, C., Laungani, P., Young, B. (1997). *Death and bereavement across cultures.* London: Routledge.